(signature) 1980

Mathematics for technologists in radiology, nuclear medicine, and radiation therapy

LEARNING RESOURCES CENTER
CLEVELAND COMMUNITY COLLEGE
137 SOUTH POST ROAD
SHELBY, NC 28150

D1200138

MATHEMATICS
for technologists
in radiology,
nuclear medicine, and
radiation therapy

STEFANO S. STEFANI, M.D.

Professor, Radiation Therapy, Rush Medical College, Chicago, Illinois;
Chief, Therapeutic Radiology Service, Veterans Administration, Edward Hines, Jr.
Hospital, Hines, Illinois; Director, Radiotherapy Department, Mt. Sinai
Hospital Medical Center, Chicago, Illinois

LINCOLN B. HUBBARD, Ph.D.

Associate Professor, Radiology and Medical Physics, Chicago Medical School,
Chicago, Ill.; Physicist Consultant, Veterans Administration, Edward Hines, Jr.
Hospital, Hines, Illinois; Mt. Sinai Hospital Medical Center and Cook County
Hospital, Chicago, Illinois; Radiation Safety Officer, Hinsdale Sanitarium and
Hospital, Hinsdale, Illinois; Partner, Fields, Griffith, and Associates, Inc.,
Glencoe, Illinois

with the technical assistance of
ERHARD SANDERS, MLL, MSLS *Deceased*
Technical Information Specialist, Midwest Research Support Center, Veterans
Administration, Edward Hines, Jr. Hospital, Hines, Illinois

with 117 illustrations

The C. V. Mosby Company
ST. LOUIS · TORONTO · LONDON   1979

21813

Copyright © 1979 by The C. V. Mosby Company

All rights reserved. No part of this book may be reproduced in any manner without written permission of the publisher.

Printed in the United States of America

The C. V. Mosby Company
11830 Westline Industrial Drive, St. Louis, Missouri 63141

Library of Congress Cataloging in Publication Data

Stefani, Stefano S   1929-
  Mathematics for technologists in radiology, nuclear medicine, and radiation therapy.

  Bibliography: p.
  Includes index.
  1. Radiology, Medical—Mathematics. I. Hubbard,
Lincoln B., 1940-   joint author. II. Sanders,
Erhard S., 1910-1979 joint author. III. Title. [DNLM:
1. Mathematics. 2. Technology, Radiologic. WN25
S812m]
R905.S83   510'.2'461   78-32110
ISBN 0-8016-4762-2

CB/CB/CB 9 8 7 6 5 4 3 2 1   02/B/220

In memory of
Erhard Sanders
whose enthusiasm, steady application,
and skill made this book possible.

Preface

Let's face it: To learn and apply radiological technology, you will need a certain amount of mathematics. There will be instances where a good foundation in mathematics will make it easier for you to understand the concepts, features, and relationships in radiology. There will be situations where mathematics is a helpful tool in making important decisions. There will indeed be circumstances where the correct application of mathematical principles may mean the difference between the success and failure of a treatment, perhaps between life and death for the patient.

In a survey conducted in 1973* we found—not quite unexpectedly—that average high school graduates throughout the country are, to put it mildly, not sufficiently prepared in mathematics for successful careers in radiological technology. This book was born out of our resolution to do something about this somewhat depressing state of affairs. It is a product of teamwork, the team consisting of a radiologist—to delineate the field; a physicist—for the laborious task of preparing the text, illustrating it with appropriate examples, and securing it with problems for you to solve; and a technical editor—to trim, to clarify, and to enhance the readability.

The book is structured to make each chapter as nearly independent of the others as possible. However, as a text it is intended to be used front to back, since techniques such as graphing (Chapter 6) will be routinely used as needed in later chapters.

The more important formulas are numbered sequentially. Those considered particularly helpful to the users of this book are boxed. The numerical examples are intended for clarification and can be skipped without loss of continuity. However, many of them illustrate connections between mathematical theorems and their applications in radiology.

The problems at the end of each chapter are divided into three sets. The first set is keyed to the numerical examples and closely parallels them. The problems in the second set are general, the type found on most mathematics tests—number problems and word problems. The third set of problems consists of objective questions.

Throughout the book we present many practical examples that refer to related disciplines, such as radiological physics. However, no attempt has

---

*Stefani, S.: Do our students know enough mathematics? Results of a survey, Rad. Technol. **46(1)**:1-5, 1974.

been made to cover all mathematical aspects of these disciplines. We have tried our best to make this book as helpful to you as possible. We hope that it will serve you well.

We acknowledge with sincere gratitude the valuable contributions made by Anna Galfredi, Professor John LeVan, and Professor Lionello Pasquini in reviewing the mathematics and making pertinent suggestions, the painstaking job of Barbara Schaff, Gloria Jaranilla, and Carol Kroc in typing the difficult text, Harold Pombert in preparing the line drawings, and the efforts of Dr. Stewart Bushong, who served as publisher's reviewer of our initial proposal and made several practical suggestions.

Stefano S. Stefani
Lincoln B. Hubbard

Contents

Mathematics for technologists in radiology, nuclear medicine, and radiation therapy

CHAPTER 1

Fundamental operations

This text is intended mainly as a practical handbook for students of radiological technology. Its purpose is to help you find answers to a variety of practical problems by the application of numerical operations. We recommend that you obtain a small electronic calculator as soon as possible.

BASIC OPERATIONS WITH SIGNED NUMBERS

Numbers can be positive, negative, or zero. Positive numbers may be written with or without a plus sign. For example, positive seven may be written as +7 or as 7. Negative numbers *must* be written with a minus sign, as with −7 for negative seven. A negative number indicates the absence of a quantity. It may also be used for distances; for instance, height is measured as a positive distance above the ground, whereas something below ground level could be said to have a negative height.

The *absolute value* of a signed number is a measure of its deviation from zero regardless of its sign. The absolute value of +3 is 3; the absolute value of −3 is also 3. The absolute value of a number is always positive, and is often denoted by vertical bars. The absolute value of −5 may be written as $|-5|$ and is equal to 5.

> **Example 1-1.** Is 3 positive or negative? What is its absolute value? Since it has no + or − sign, it is assumed to be positive. Its absolute value is its positive value, which is 3.
>
> **Example 1-2.** What is the absolute value of −9? The absolute value of −9 is 9 or $|-9| = 9$.

In arithmetic operations involving two numbers the results have two properties: the magnitude, or absolute value, of the result, and the sign, which tells us whether the result is positive or negative.

ADDITION OF SIGNED NUMBERS. To add two numbers with the same sign, one adds their absolute values. The result, or sum, will carry the common sign. For example, 3 plus 5 is 8, and −4 plus −5 is −9.

> **Example 1-3.** Add −7 and −2. The sum will have the absolute value $7 + 2 = 9$ and the sign will be negative. Hence the sum is −9.

To add two numbers with opposite signs, one finds the difference between the absolute values of the two numbers. The sum will carry the sign of the number with the greater absolute value.

> **Example 1-4.** Add 3 and −5. The difference between 5 and 3 is 2. The sign of the sum must be negative, since 5 is greater than 3. Hence the result is −2.

Order of signed numbers in addition. Signed numbers are usually added in the order in which they are given. For example, in 3 + 4 + 9 the 3 and 4 are added first; 9 is then added to the result to give the overall sum of 16.

In addition operations such as 3 + 4, we can proceed in any order; the result is always the same. This can be written formally by reordering the elements of the sum, called "addends," into a new order:

$$3 + 4 = 4 + 3$$

The possibility of reordering addends is stated in the *commutative law of addition*. This law may seem trivial, but it will be a useful concept in later developments, particularly in algebra.

Another aspect of addition is that the subgroups of a series of addends can be rearranged. For example, to add 4 + 5 + 6, 4 + 5 can be grouped first, and the 6 then added to the result: 4 + 5 + 6 = 9 + 6 = 15. Or 5 + 6 can be grouped first and the 4 added to that result: 4 + 5 + 6 = 4 + 11 = 15. The sum will always be the same. This possibility of rearranging subgroups of a sum is stated in the *associative law of addition*. A useful application of this law is shown in the following example.

> **Example 1-5.** Add 83 + 40 + 17 + 160. This is most conveniently done by adding 83 and 17 to equal 100 and 40 and 160 to equal 200. Using this grouping and the commutative law, we have 100 + 200, or 300.

If an operation contains both positive and negative numbers, it helps to combine all positive numbers in one group and all negative numbers in another.

SUBTRACTION OF SIGNED NUMBERS. The subtraction of 4 from 7 is written as 7 − 4. In this expression, 7 is called the "minuend," 4 is called "subtrahend," and the result is called the "difference." The subtraction of 4 from 7 is the same as the addition of 7 and −4, that is, subtraction can be conceived of as addition with the subtrahend given as a negative value.

> **Example 1-6.** Subtract 2 from −3. This will equal the addition of −3 and −2 or −3 − 2, which is −5.

If the subtrahend itself is negative, we are taking away a negative amount. This is equivalent to adding a positive amount; the elimination of a loss or a debt is a positive gain. Hence the subtraction of a negative quantity is equal to the addition of the absolute value of a quantity. For example, 3 minus -2 is equal to $3 + 2$ or 5.

> **Example 1-7.** What is the result of subtracting -5 from -7? The expression $-7 - (-5)$ is equal to $-7 + 5 = -2$.

MULTIPLICATION OF SIGNED NUMBERS. Multiplication of signed numbers yields a *product*, the absolute value of which is equal to the product of the absolute values of the factors. The sign of the product is positive if both factors are positive or if both factors are negative. Thus $-3 \times -5 = |-3| \times |-5| = 15$. But if one factor is positive and one is negative, the product is negative. For example, $+3 \times -4 = -|3 \times 4| = -12$.

> **Example 1-8.** What is the product of -2×4? Its absolute value is 8; the sign is negative because -2 is negative and 4 is positive. The answer is -8.

Note that the sign for multiplication may be "$\times$" or a dot higher than a period. Computers often use an asterisk, and in those cases where the sign can be left out, multiplication is always the implied operation.

The order of the factors in a product is irrelevant. For example:

$$3 \times -2 = -2 \times 3$$

This is stated in the *commutative law of multiplication*. There is also an *associative law of multiplication*. (See later discussion of grouping and parentheses).

DIVISION OF SIGNED NUMBERS. A division, say 12 divided by 3, is represented in one of two notations: 12/3 or $12 \div 3$. In this example, 12 is the *dividend*, 3 is the *divisor*, and the result, 4, is the *quotient* (or the *ratio*).

The rules of division are very similar to those of multiplication. The absolute value of a quotient is equal to the quotient of the absolute value of the dividend and the absolute value of the divisor. The quotient is positive if the dividend and the divisor have the same sign; if one is positive and the other is negative, the quotient is negative.

> **Example 1-9.** What is the quotient $-28 \div 7$? The absolute value of the quotient is $28 \div 7$, or 4. The sign is negative, since -28 is negative and 7 is positive. Hence the answer is -4.

> **Example 1-10.** What is the quotient $-6 \div -3$? The magnitude of the quotient is 2 and the sign is positive. The quotient is 2.

Note that there is no commutative or associative law for division. For instance, $12 \div 3$ is *not* equal to $3 \div 12$.

FRACTIONS

The numbers with which we have operated thus far are called *whole numbers*. They are sufficient in many situations, but it is frequently necessary to deal with a part or *fraction* of a whole number. There are several types of fractions: common fractions, decimal fractions, and percents.

COMMON FRACTIONS. When we divide a whole into a certain number of equal parts, each of these parts is represented by a one "over" that number. This representation is called a fraction. For example, $^1/_7$ is a fraction representing one of seven equal parts into which the whole quantity was divided.

> **Example 1-11.** Express 1 hour as a fraction of a day. Since there are 24 hours in a day, each hour is $^1/_{24}$ of a day.

If a number of equal portions are added, this number appears as the dividend, with the total number of equal portions as the divisor. For example, if an item is divided into seven parts, three of these parts are represented as $^3/_7$. In this division, 3 is the dividend and 7 is the divisor. However, the terminology is different; the dividend is called the *numerator* and divisor is called the *denominator*.

> **Example 1-12.** If an object is divided into five parts, what fraction represents two of these parts? The fraction is $^2/_5$.

For every fraction, there is, theoretically, an infinite number of other fractions of equal value. For instance, one half hour can be represented as $^1/_2$ if we consider the hour divided into two equal parts. If the hour is divided into four equal parts (quarters of an hour), a half hour is two quarter hours or $^2/_4$. If the hour is divided into minutes, a half hour is $^{30}/_{60}$. These fractions are all equal:

$$^1/_2 = {}^2/_4 = {}^{30}/_{60}$$

Which of these forms we actually use depends on the situation. The most frequently used form is the one involving the smallest whole numbers. In our example this is $^1/_2$.

Fractions can be simplified by *factoring*. Many whole numbers are the product of two other whole numbers. For example, in the equation $24 = 6 \times 4$, 6 and 4 are factors of 24. Numbers that cannot be broken into two or more factors (other than 1) are called *primes*. Examples of primes are 2, 3, 5, 7, and 11. The numbers 4, 6, 8, 10, and 12 are not primes. All whole numbers except primes can be expressed as the product of prime factors ($24 = 2 \times 2 \times 2 \times 3$ in prime factors).

Example 1-13. Express 42 in prime factors. $42 = 2 \times 3 \times 7$.

A fraction can be simplified if the numerator and denominator have some common factor. For example, in the fraction $^{30}\!/_{60}$, $30 = 5 \times 6$ and $60 = 5 \times 12$; the number 5 is a common factor and can be canceled (this operation will be explained later): $\dfrac{30}{60} = \dfrac{5 \times 6}{5 \times 12} = \dfrac{\cancel{5} \times 6}{\cancel{5} \times 12} = \dfrac{6}{12}$

Example 1-14. Reduce $^{6}\!/_{12}$ to its simplest form. Six is a common factor; thus $\dfrac{6}{12} = \dfrac{6 \times 1}{6 \times 2} = \dfrac{1}{2}$.

A fraction is in its simplest form if there is no common factor when the numbers are expressed as products of primes.

Example 1-15. Is $^{25}\!/_{98}$ in its simplest form? In prime factors this is $\dfrac{5 \times 5}{2 \times 7 \times 7}$. Since there are no common prime factors, this is the simplest form.

Another useful manipulation of a fraction is taking the *inverse*. This amounts to flipping the fraction over. Thus the inverse of $-\dfrac{3}{5}$ is $-\dfrac{5}{3}$; note that fractions can be negative or have a magnitude greater than 1.

Fractions can be added, subtracted, multiplied, or divided. The result of any of these operations will be a fraction. All such operations obey the same rules as those with whole numbers in the previous section.

If fractions are to be added, their denominators must be the same. The result will be a fraction with the same denominator and a numerator that will be the sum of the numerators of the single fractions. For example, $^{1}\!/_{5}$ plus $^{3}\!/_{5}$ is $^{4}\!/_{5}$:

$$\frac{1}{5} + \frac{3}{5} = \frac{1 + 3}{5} = \frac{4}{5}$$

Example 1-16. Add $^{3}\!/_{4}$ and $-^{1}\!/_{4}$. Since the denominators are both the same, this can be added as $\dfrac{3}{4} + \dfrac{-1}{4} = \dfrac{3 - 1}{4} = \dfrac{2}{4}$. The result is $^{2}\!/_{4}$ or, by factoring and canceling out the common factor 2, $^{1}\!/_{2}$.

Suppose the denominators of the fractions to be added are not the same, for instance, $^{1}\!/_{3}$ and $^{1}\!/_{2}$. It is then necessary to modify one or both so as to have equal denominators. This is done by reversing the factoring used earlier to simplify a fraction. By multiplying numerator and denominator by the factor 2 we can change $\frac{1}{3}$ to $\frac{2}{6}$: $\frac{1}{3} = \frac{1 \times 2}{3 \times 2} = \frac{2}{6}$; $\frac{1}{2}$ is changed to $\frac{3}{6}$ by using the factor 3. With these changes, $\frac{1}{3} + \frac{1}{2}$ becomes $\frac{2}{6} + \frac{3}{6}$. In this latter form, we can add to obtain $\frac{5}{6}$. We were able to add $\frac{1}{3}$ and $\frac{1}{2}$ after we had changed these fractions to equivalent ones with a *common denominator,* in this case 6. The easiest common denominator to find is the product of the two denominators.

Example 1-17. Add the two fractions $\frac{1}{7}$ and $\frac{5}{9}$. The smallest common denominator is $7 \times 9 = 63$. The fraction $\frac{1}{7}$ is equal to $\frac{1 \times 9}{7 \times 9} = \frac{9}{63}$ and $\frac{5}{9}$ is equal to $\frac{5 \times 7}{9 \times 7} = \frac{35}{63}$. Thus the sum is equal to $\frac{9 + 35}{63} = \frac{44}{63}$.

After addition or another operation involving common fractions, it is often possible to simplify the result by factoring.

If we want to add whole numbers to fractions, we write the whole number in the form of a fraction with 1 as the denominator and the number as the numerator. For example, we can write 27 as $\frac{27}{1}$, since the division of 27 by 1 will equal 27.

Example 1-18. A certain technician's time is computed in half days. If he works two full days and one half day during a week, how many half days is this? Here we add 2 and $\frac{1}{2}$ as follows: $2 + \frac{1}{2} = \frac{2}{1} + \frac{1}{2} = \frac{2 \times 2}{1 \times 2} + \frac{1}{2} = \frac{4}{2} + \frac{1}{2} = \frac{5}{2}$. The technician is credited with five half days.

If one or both of the fractions are negative, the signs are normally associated with the numerators. The addition of the numerators follows the rule for addition of signed numbers.

Example 1-19. During one week, $\frac{1}{2}$ curie (Ci) of a certain radionuclide is received from a supplier. During the same week, approximately $\frac{2}{3}$ Ci either decays or is used. What is the net change in amount of radionuclide? Additions are considered as positive and losses as negative. The change is $\frac{1}{2} - \frac{2}{3}$. This is: $\frac{1}{2} - \frac{2}{3} = \frac{1 \times 3}{2 \times 3} - \frac{2 \times 2}{3 \times 2}$

$= \frac{3}{6} - \frac{4}{6} = \frac{3 - 4}{6} = -\frac{1}{6}$. Hence there is a loss of $\frac{1}{6}$ Ci.

Subtraction of fractions follows the same rule as subtraction of signed whole numbers. It is done by adding the first fraction to the negative of the second fraction. Again, the subtraction of a negative quantity is the same as the addition of a positive quantity.

In the multiplication of two fractions the numerators and denominators are multiplied separately. For example, $\frac{2}{3} \times \frac{4}{7} = \frac{2 \times 4}{3 \times 7} = \frac{8}{21}$.

Example 1-20. At 1 cm from a 1 mg source of radium (^{226}Ra) the exposure rate is $8\frac{1}{4}$ roentgens/hour (R/hr). At 3 cm the exposure will be $\frac{1}{9}$ of this. What is the exposure rate at 3 cm from this 1 mg source? First, add the 8 to the $\frac{1}{4}$ to obtain $\frac{8}{1} + \frac{1}{4} = \frac{8 \times 4}{4} + \frac{1}{4} = \frac{32}{4} + \frac{1}{4} = \frac{33}{4}$ R/hr and then multiply by $\frac{1}{9}$ to obtain $\frac{1}{9} \times \frac{33}{4} = \frac{1 \times 33}{9 \times 4} = \frac{33}{36}$, which can be simplified to $\frac{11}{12}$ R/hr.

Division by a whole number is the same as multiplication by a fraction with 1 in the numerator and the number in the denominator. For example, multiplication by $\frac{1}{5}$ is equal to division by 5; $\frac{1}{5}$ is the inverse of 5. Division of one fraction by another is performed by multiplying the dividend by the inverse of the divisor. For example, $\frac{3}{4} \div \frac{2}{3} = \frac{3}{4} \times \frac{3}{2} = \frac{9}{8}$.

Example 1-21. In a radiology lab, $^{17}/_2$ dosages are to be arranged in amounts of $\frac{1}{3}$ dose each. How many $\frac{1}{3}$ doses will there be? The result is the quotient of $^{17}/_2 \div \frac{1}{3}$: This is $\frac{^{17}/_2}{^{1}/_3} = \frac{17}{2} \times \frac{3}{1} = \frac{51}{2}$, or $25\frac{1}{2}$ such doses.

DECIMAL REPRESENTATION OF FRACTIONS. There are many drawbacks in using common fractions for calculations that involve fractional parts of whole numbers. Probably the most serious is the fact that common fractions are not represented by electronic calculators and computers because two whole numbers are required to represent the fractional portion.

One way to avoid this problem is to use a standard or implied denominator. This is done with *decimals,* in which all the denominators are powers of 10 and the position of the decimal point tells us which power is used.

A well-known decimal representation is that used for money. For example, we represent 25¢ or $1/4$ dollar as $0.25. The 0.25 is a representation of $^{25}/_{100}$. In decimals the fractional part of a number is to the right of the decimal point and the whole number is to the left. If there is one digit to the right, the implied denominator is 10; with two digits to the right, it is 100; with three digits, it is 1,000; and so on.

> **Example 1-22.** A rod measures 1.125 inches. Express this as a whole plus a fractional part in common fraction form. The whole is, of course, 1. The fraction is $^{125}/_{1000}$.
>
> This can be factored as follows: $\dfrac{125}{1000} = \dfrac{5 \times 5 \times 5}{5 \times 5 \times 5 \times 8}$
>
> Hence $1.125 = 1^{1}/_{8}$.

This example illustrates the method of converting decimal fractions to common fractions. The fractional portion is represented as the numerator, and the appropriate power of 10 is represented as the denominator.

The conversion from common fractions to decimals requires more work, except for some simpler values. Among these we have already seen that $1/4$ is equal to 0.25. Since $1/2$ can be represented as $^{5}/_{10}$, it has the decimal representation of 0.5. Placing a zero to the left of the decimal point in numbers less than one is optional, but is recommended to call attention to the decimal point.

Fractions such as $1/3$ cannot be turned into a decimal by the preceding procedure because there is no power of 10 of which 3 is an exact factor. For the conversion of $1/3$ to a decimal we divide 3 into 1.0000 . . . (as many zeros as we wish):

$$
\begin{array}{r}
0.333 \\
3\,\overline{)\,1.000} \\
\underline{9} \\
10 \\
\underline{9} \\
10 \\
\underline{9} \\
1
\end{array}
$$

In this process the decimal point of the result (the quotient) is placed directly above the decimal point in the dividend. There is no decimal point in the divisor. The decimal representation for $1/3$ is an example of a *repeating decimal,* in which one or more digits form a group that repeats itself as more zeros are added to the dividend. The fraction $1/4$ is a *terminating decimal,* as only two zeros are required to the right of the decimal. All common fractions have either a terminating or a repeating decimal representation. When dealing with fractions that have repeating decimal representations, how many digits

are we to write, since theoretically they never end? Mathematicians some-
times use a line over or under the repeating group, as in the expression $\frac{1}{3} = 0.3\overline{3}$, to indicate this repetition. The practical limitations of accuracy are discussed in Chapter 2.

Example 1-23. Express two days as a decimal fraction of one week.
Carrying out the division:

$$
\begin{array}{r}
0.285714 \\
7\,)\overline{2.0} \\
1\,4 \\
\hline
60 \\
56 \\
\hline
40 \\
35 \\
\hline
50 \\
49 \\
\hline
10 \\
7 \\
\hline
30 \\
28 \\
\hline
2
\end{array}
$$

Thus $\frac{2}{7}$ is 0.285714.

The conversion from common fractions to decimals can be carried out by
division on an electronic calculator or a slide rule.

Mathematical operations with decimals are easy. For additions or subtractions in the decimal representation, it is important to line up the numbers so
that the decimal points are in line. For example, we write:

$$
\begin{array}{r}
0.25 \\
+0.2857
\end{array}
$$

If we wish, we can add trailing zeros to any decimal. In our example we might
write:

$$
\begin{array}{r}
0.2500 \\
+0.2857
\end{array}
$$

The sum or difference is then written with the decimal point in the same
column. In our example:

$$
\begin{array}{r}
0.2500 \\
+0.2857 \\
\hline
0.5357
\end{array}
$$

Example 1-24. You have 1.342 millicuries (mCi) of ^{99m}Tc bound on microspheres. If you remove 0.15 mCi, how much is left? This is found by subtracting 0.15 from 1.342. We write:

$$
\begin{array}{r}
1.342 \\
-0.150 \\
\hline
1.192
\end{array}
$$

Thus there are 1.192 mCi left.

For multiplication, we ignore the decimal point in the operation itself and place it in the product as many digits to the left as there are decimal places in the operation. For example, 3.75×0.2 is first multiplied as 375×2 to give 750. The decimal point is placed to the left of three digits, since 3.75 has two decimals places and 0.2 has one. Thus $3.75 \times 0.2 = 0.750$.

Example 1-25. In one month the strength of a ^{60}Co source will decay to about 0.989 of its initial amount. If a source has 2,743 Ci at the beginning of the month, what will it have at the end of the month? The amount will be $0.989 \times 2,743$; $989 \times 2,743 = 2,712,827$. With the decimal point properly placed, the result is 2,712.827 Ci.

Division of decimals is carried out by making the denominator a whole number. This is done by multiplying both the divisor and the dividend by the appropriate factor. For example, $3.75 \div 0.4$ can be written as $\dfrac{3.75}{0.4}$, which is equal to $\dfrac{3.75 \times 10}{0.4 \times 10} = \dfrac{37.5}{4}$. To eliminate the decimal point in 0.4, we multiply by 10. This effectively "moves" the decimal point one place to the right. We do the same with the dividend. Thus in an operational sense the first step of division is to move the decimal point of both divisor and dividend to the right by as many places as there are decimal places in the divisor. The decimal point of the quotient is then written over the decimal point of the modified dividend. In our example:

$$
\begin{array}{r}
9.375 \\
4\,\overline{)\,37.5} \\
36 \\
\hline
1\,5 \\
1\,2 \\
\hline
30 \\
28 \\
\hline
20 \\
20
\end{array}
$$

Example 1-26. Normal atmospheric pressure is 760 mm of mercury (mm Hg). What is the ratio of 757 mm Hg to normal atmospheric pressure? The ratio 757/760 with an implied decimal point after the last 7 in the numerator. The result of the division $760\overline{)757}$ is 0.996 to three decimal places.

PERCENTS. Percent, abbreviated from the Latin phrase *per centum*, means per hundred, and it can be represented by a fraction whose denominator is 100. Thus 10 percent, or 10%, is equal to $^{10}/_{100}$ ($^{1}/_{10}$ in simplified form).

> **Example 1-27.** What is 25% expressed as a common fraction? It is $^{25}/_{100}$ or, simplified, $^{1}/_{4}$.

Although percents can be converted to common fractions, it is even easier to convert them to decimals. Arithmetical operations with percents are usually performed in decimals. Because the implied denominator for percent is 100, its decimal equivalent has the decimal point two places to the left. Thus 3% of a certain amount is equal to 0.03, and 15% is equal to 0.15.

> **Example 1-28.** Express 50% as a decimal and as a fraction. The decimal will be 0.50 or 0.5; the fraction will be $^{50}/_{100}$ or $^{1}/_{2}$.

> **Example 1-29.** Express 0.65 as percent. This is 65%.

Percents are mainly used for values between 1 and 100. Beyond this range, care must be taken when interpreting their value. For example, 250% is equal to 2.5 as a decimal, and $^{1}/_{2}$%, which equals 0.5%, is equal to 0.005 in decimal representation.

Percents are also used to express changes. A phrase such as "increased by 10%" means that the final value is equal to the initial value plus 10% of *that* value. We obtain the 10% by multiplying the initial value by 0.1 and the final value by multiplying the initial value by 1.1.

> **Example 1-30.** To increase a quantity by 25%, by how much must we multiply it? Since 25% is 0.25, we should multiply by 1.25.

If our initial quantity is decreased by a certain percentage, then the multiplication factor is 1.0 minus the decrease as a decimal. Thus a 25% decrease is obtained by multiplying by 0.75.

> **Example 1-31.** Every hour, a source of technetium (^{99m}Tc) will decay in strength by 11%. By what factor should we multiply an initial activity of ^{99m}Tc to find its activity after one hour? Since the decrease is 11%, the factor should be 0.89.

If we have the value after the change and wish to find the initial amount, we divide by the factor as just determined.

> **Example 1-32.** At 7 AM a vial of ^{99m}Tc contains 50 mCi. What was its activity at 6 AM, when it was delivered? For a one hour change, we divide by the factor from example 1-31, which is 0.89. Thus the activity at 6 AM was $^{50}/_{0.89}$ = 56 mCi.

GROUPING AND PARENTHESES

When a problem requires more than one operation, there may be some uncertainty as to which operation comes first. For example, in the expression $2 + 3 \div 5$, are we to add $2 + 3$ first to obtain $5 \div 5$ or are we to divide 3 by 5 first to obtain $2 + 0.6$?

PRIORITY OF OPERATIONS. To eliminate any ambiguity, mathematicians have established a priority of operations that calls for *multiplication and division before addition and subtraction*. Thus in the example $2 + 3 \div 5$, the division must be performed to give us $2 + 0.6 = 2.6$ (or $2 \, ^3/_5$). This must never be reversed. The general rule, if there are no symbols of grouping, is to perform all multiplications *or* divisions *first*, whichever is met first from left to right, *then* to perform all additions *or* subtractions, whichever comes first from left to right.

> **Example 1-33.** Express $3 \div 4 + 2$ in decimals. Here the division is the first operation carried out: $3 \div 4 + 2 = 0.75 + 2$. Next, the addition yields 2.75.

PARENTHESES. If we want to add two numbers and then divide the sum by a third number, we *must* indicate that the normal order of priorities is not to be followed. We do this by enclosing the operation to be performed first in parentheses. For example, if we write $(2 + 3) \div 5$, the addition is to be done first. Operations in parentheses take priority over others. When more than one operation is enclosed in parentheses, the grouped operations can be performed in any desired order.

> **Example 1-34.** The conversion of temperature in Fahrenheit (T_f) to Celsius temperature (T_c) can be given by the following formula:
>
> $$T_c = (T_f - 32) \times 5 \div 9$$
>
> Which operation is performed first? The first operation performed is the one in parentheses, subtraction.

When more than one pair of parentheses are required in a single expression, it is best to use different forms, such as brackets and braces. Thus an expression might be written as follows:

$$\left\{\left[(2+4) \div 5\right] + \left[6 + 1 \div 3\right]\right\} \div 5$$

In this case the priority goes to those parenthetical pairs that do not enclose any other parenthetical phrases.

> **Example 1-35.** In the expression just given, which operation must be done first? The addition in the first parentheses $(2 + 4)$ or the division in the second pair of brackets $(1 \div 3)$ must be done before any other operation.

On computers and certain larger calculators, parentheses are available and invaluable, since expressions are restricted to a single line. However, care in their use is needed because only one form is available. The computer or calculator also expects all parentheses to be in pairs, and will reject expressions that do not have an equal number of left and right parentheses. The previous expression would appear on a computer as $(((2 + 4) \div 5) + (6 + 1 \div 3)) \div 5$.

When parentheses are used, it is customary to drop the multiplication sign. For example, $3(2 - 4)$ means 3 times the difference of 2 and 4, and $(4 + 2)(3 - 1)$ is the same as $4 + 2$ times $3 - 1$. For the expression in parentheses, the minus sign implies multiplication by -1. Thus, $-(2 - 3)$ is equal to $-2 + 3$; both signs within the parentheses are changed by the minus sign in front. In an expression such as $3 + (5 \div 9)$ the parentheses are "redundant," since $3 + 5 \div 9$ is the same. Redundant parentheses are not wrong. They may be deleted if desired or inserted for emphasis. For example, we could illustrate the associative law by the following example:

$$(4 + 5) + 6 = 4 + (5 + 6)$$

DISTRIBUTIVE LAW. A law pertaining to addition *and* multiplication is called the *distributive law*. It relates to the product of a sum. For example:

$$3(2 + 4) = 3 \times 2 + 3 \times 4$$

That is, the product of the factor and the sum is equal to the sum of the products of the factor and the individual addends.

The distributive law can be used in reverse. If we have the sum of two addends with a common factor (for example, $20 + 75$, which have 5 as a common factor), we can *factor out* so that we obtain the form of the distributive law. Thus $20 + 75 = 5 \times 4 + 5 \times 15 = 5(4 + 15)$. A corresponding distributive law for division exists, since division by a number is equivalent to multiplication by the inverse of that number. Thus $(5 + 2) \div 4 = 5 \div 4 + 2 \div 4$.

The use of parentheses and the distributive law are much more important in algebra, where the quantities in an operation do not necessarily have a known numerical value. This will be discussed further in Chapter 3.

POWERS AND ROOTS OF NUMBERS

POWER REPRESENTATION. If we want to express 384 in prime factors, we can write it as $2 \times 2 \times 2 \times 2 \times 2 \times 2 \times 2 \times 3$. The representation is correct, but we might get tired of writing the seven 2's. By utilizing the power notation, we can write the seven 2's as 2^7. The raised 7 is called the power or *exponent*. On computers 2^7 is printed on a single line as 2**7. The expression is read as "two to the seventh power" or "two to the seventh."

> **Example 1-36.** Write 10,000 as a power of 10. The number 10,000 is equal to $10 \times 10 \times 10 \times 10$ or 10^4.

Certain powers have special names. The *square* is the second power. Thus "4 squared" or "the square or 4" is $4^2 = 16$. The *cube* is the third power.

> **Example 1-37.** What is the cube of 7? It is $7^3 = 7 \times 7 \times 7 = 49 \times 7 = 343$.

The multiplication of two powers of the same number, for example $2^3 \times 2^4$, is very simple. To multiply two powers of the same number, we add the exponents. Here, three factors of 2 are multiplied by four factors of 2, a total of seven factors of 2. Thus $2^3 \times 2^4 = 2^{(3+4)} = 2^7$.

NEGATIVE POWERS. If two powers of the same number are divided, the power of the quotient is the difference of the exponents. For example, $5^4 \div 5^2 = \dfrac{5 \times 5 \times 5 \times 5}{5 \times 5} = 5 \times 5 = 5^2$, or $5^4 \div 5^2 = 5^{(4-2)} = 5^2$.

> **Example 1-38.** What is $6^5 \div 6^3$? This is $6^{(5-3)} = 6^2$.

This rule for division leads us to some interesting properties of the power notation. First, consider the example $3^3 \div 3^2$. By our rule, this must equal 3^1. If the powers are expanded, this is $\dfrac{3 \times 3 \times 3}{3 \times 3} = 3$. Thus we see that $3^1 = 3$.

In general terms, any number raised to the first power is the number itself. Consider another special case, $5^2 \div 5^2$. This is $5^{(2-2)} = 5^0$ by our rule for dividing exponents. It is also $\dfrac{5 \times 5}{5 \times 5} = 1$. In general terms, any number to the zero power is 1.

A third special case of division is the situation in which the power of the divisor exceeds the power of the dividend. For example, $2^5 \div 2^7$. The rule for division in this case would give $2^5 \div 2^7 = 2^{-2}$. Expanding the powers gives

$$\frac{2 \times 2 \times 2 \times 2 \times 2}{2 \times 2 \times 2 \times 2 \times 2 \times 2 \times 2} = \frac{1}{2 \times 2}.$$ We see that $2^{-2} = \frac{1}{2 \times 2}$, or $\frac{1}{2^2}$. A negative exponent represents the inverse of a power or a power in the denominator.

Example 1-39. Represent 0.001 as a power of 10. This decimal is equal to $\frac{1}{10 \times 10 \times 10}$, or 10^{-3}.

Some of the negative powers have special names. The "inverse of" means the power -1. The "inverse square" is the power -2, and the "inverse cube" is the power -3.

FRACTIONAL POWERS AND ROOTS. In the expression $3^2 = 9$, we can call 9 the square of 3 or we can call 3 the *square root* of 9. The square root of a number is that value which, when multiplied by itself, gives the number. The square of a whole number is always a whole number, but the square root frequently is not; the square root of 2 is approximately 1.414 (not a repeating decimal). The square root is usually represented by the radical sign, as in $\sqrt{2}$. The cube root is indicated by the radical and a 3 raised above it, as in $\sqrt[3]{2}$.

WORD PROBLEMS

For much routine work the general form of the manipulation is well known, and the whole effort of obtaining a correct answer is directed at the arithmetic. Nonstandard problems, however, pose a very different situation. With these the choice of operation is as important as the correct completion of the opera-

Table 1

Some key words in mathematical word problems

Word	Addition	Subtraction	Multiplication	Division
And	*			
Balance		*		
By			*	
Decrease		*	0	
Difference		*		
Each			*	0
Factor			*	
Fraction of				*
Group of				*
Less		*	0	
More		*		
Percent of			0	*
Plus	*			
Of			*	
Together	*			
Total	*			
With	*			

* = likely.
0 = possible, but not very likely.

tion. Obviously, if we should multiply, addition is not likely to yield the correct answer.

SIGNIFICANT ELEMENTS. In word problems we are usually given the necessary elements and an indication of how the elements are to be handled. The key to the operation expected is usually contained in the words linking the numerical elements. For example, if a question is phrased "one half of 600 people," the word "of" indicates multiplication by $\frac{1}{2}$. Some common key words and their significance are listed in Table 1 on p. 15. This list is neither exhaustive nor infallible.

CHAPTER REVIEW

1. What is the absolute value of a negative number?
2. Of the four basic operations, which one does not have a commutative law? Is the sum of two negative numbers positive or negative?
3. Is the product of two negative numbers positive or negative?
4. What is the numerator of a common fraction?
5. What is a common denominator?
6. What is the inverse of a fraction?
7. How is the decimal converted to a common fraction?
8. How are decimal numbers added?
9. What is the relationship between percents and decimals?
10. Which operations have priority?
11. How do parentheses reorder the priorities of an operation?
12. What notation is used to indicate a power?
13. What is the meaning of a negative power?

PROBLEMS

At the end of each chapter we present three groups of problems. The first closely parallels the examples in the text. The second contains more general problems that may draw on any of the material we have discussed thus far. In the last group, we pose objective questions on this material. Selected answers appear in Appendix B.

Problems paralleling chapter examples

The example number is given in parentheses following the question number.

1. **(1-1)** Is -7 positive or negative?
2. **(1-2)** What is the absolute value of -1?
3. **(1-3)** Add -1 and -3.
4. **(1-4)** Add -4 and 7.
5. **(1-6)** Subtract -2 from 3.
6. **(1-7)** Subtract -4 from -3.
7. **(1-8)** What is the product of -4 and -5?
8. **(1-9)** What is the quotient of $-25 \div 5$?
9. **(1-10)** What is the quotient of $18 \div -2$?
10. **(1-11)** Express one day as a fraction of a week.
11. **(1-12)** A quantity is divided into seven equal groups. What fraction represents four of these groups?
12. **(1-13)** Express 36 in prime factors.
13. **(1-14)** Reduce $\frac{24}{64}$ to its simplest form.
14. **(1-15)** Is $\frac{15}{42}$ in its simplest form?
15. **(1-16)** Add $-\frac{1}{7}$ and $\frac{3}{7}$.
16. **(1-17)** Add $\frac{2}{3}$ and $\frac{1}{4}$.
17. **(1-18)** How many quarter hours are there in $2\frac{1}{4}$ hours?
18. **(1-20)** A certain dose of ^{99m}Tc is $\frac{2}{5}$ mCi (0.4 mCi). After twelve hours it will be $\frac{1}{4}$ of this. How much will this be in mCi?
19. **(1-22)** Express 0.75 as a common fraction.
20. **(1-23)** Express $\frac{4}{5}$ as a decimal.
21. **(1-24)** The timer on a certain therapy unit indicates 1,242.6 hours of operation at the beginning of the week. If the unit is used for 1.2 additional hours, what will the new reading be?
22. **(1-25)** In one year, a radioactive cesium

(^{137}Cs) source will decay by a factor of 0.98. At the end of a year, what will be the strength of a source that started as 15 mCi?

23. **(1-26)** One Fahrenheit degree is $5/9$ of a Celsius degree. Express this as a repeating decimal.

24. **(1-27)** What is 60% expressed as a common fraction?

25. **(1-28)** Express 12.5% as a decimal and as a common fraction.

26. **(1-29)** Express 0.7 as a percent.

27. **(1-30)** If the use of radiological procedures is increasing by 10% per year, what is the multiplicative change for one year?

28. **(1-31)** A ^{137}Cs source decays at a rate of approximately 1% every six months, that is, it decreases in strength by 1% every six months. By what factor should we multiply the present source strength to find its value in six months?

29. **(1-33)** The conversion of temperature in Celsius (T_c) to temperature in Fahrenheit (T_f) can be given by the following formula:

$$T_f = \frac{9}{5} T_c + 32$$

Of the operations indicated or implied (multiplication, division, and addition), which is performed *last*?

30. **(1-34)** To convert gauge pressure (pressure above atmospheric, P_g) measured in atmospheres (atm), to absolute pressure (P_a) measured in centimeters of mercury (mm Hg) we could use the formula:

$$P_a = 760(1 + P_g)$$

Which operation is carried out first?

31. **(1-36)** Express 1,000,000 as a power of 10.

32. **(1-37)** What is the square of 9?

33. **(1-38)** What is $5^3 \div 5^2$?

34. **(1-39)** What is 0.1 as a power of 10?

Problems related to this chapter

35. Carry out the operations indicated.
    a. $5 - (-3) =$
    b. $12 \div (-3) =$
    c. $4(-2) =$
    d. $-9 + (-2) =$

36. Carry out the operations indicated. Express the results as single common fractions.

a. $5 \div 17 =$
b. $1/3 + 1/2 =$
c. $2/3 \times 1/5 =$
d. $1/4 \div 1/3 =$

37. Carry out the operations indicated. Express the answers as decimals.
    a. $9 \div 25 =$
    b. $1.27 - 3.62 =$
    c. $1.1 \times 3.1 =$
    d. $3.0 \div 1.2 =$

38. Express $7/8$ as a decimal and as a percent.

39. What is the value of 30% of 40?

40. Which is the largest: 10%, $1/8$, or 0.11?

41. Calculate 1.2^3 and express it as a decimal without the power.

42. The "percent backscatter" is the increase in radiation dose resulting from radiation scattered by material behind the region of interest. This increase can be described by the multiplicative "backscatter factor." If a certain situation has a backscatter factor of 1.1, what is the percent backscatter?

43. The exposure from a point source of radium is decreased by 2% for each 0.1 mm of platinum (Pt) filtration added beyond 0.5 mm. What is the multiplicative factor for 0.75 mm Pt?

44. What is 1,024 expressed as a power of 2?

45. Express 10^{-6} as a common fraction.

46. If $5^2 = 25$, what is $\sqrt{25}$?

Objective questions

Indicate the correct answer.

47. The value of $(-1/2)^2$ is
    a. 4   d. $-2/4$
    b. $1/2$ e. 0.25
    c. -1

48. The quantity $\sqrt{49}$ is
    a. 7   d. 2,401
    b. 10   e. 32.9
    c. 13

49. The number that is 25% more than 8 is
    a. 2   d. 10
    b. 4   e. 12
    c. 8

50. The sum of $1/2$ and $-1/3$ is
    a. $1/6$ d. $4/6$
    b. $2/6$ e. $5/6$
    c. $3/6$

51. The value of $(1/4 + 2/5) \div 1/10$ is
    a. $3/2$ d. $10/9$
    b. $2/13$ e. $6 1/2$
    c. $9/10$

52. The sum of 2.27 and 1.1 is
    a. 3.37   d. 2.16
    b. 2,497   e. 1.17
    c. 2.38
53. The fraction $^2/_3$ expressed as a percent is approximately
    a. 5%   d. 67%
    b. 6%   e. 150%
    c. 23%
54. The fraction $\dfrac{2^6}{2^3}$ is equal to

    a. 8   d. $^1/_4$
    b. 4   e. $^1/_8$
    c. 1
55. The value of $(-2) - (-3) \div (6 - 2)$ is equal to
    a. $^1/_8$ d. $-^5/_8$
    b. $^1/_4$ e. $-^5/_4$
    c. 1
56. One tenth of 350 is *not* equal to
    a. $^{350}/_{10}$ d. $\sqrt[10]{350}$
    b. 35   e. 0.1 of 350
    c. 10% of 350

57. The inverse of 0.125 is
    a. 125   d. 1.25
    b. 12.5   e. 0.008
    c. 8
58. The expression 3(7) can also be written as
    a. 3 + 7   d. 3 ÷ 7
    b. 3 − 7   e. $\sqrt[3]{7}$
    c. 3 × 7
59. The fraction $^2/_5$ is *not* equal to
    a. 40%   d. 0.40
    b. $^4/_{10}$ e. 4%
    c. $^{10}/_{25}$
60. One inch is what fraction of a foot?
    a. $^1/_{12}$ d. $^{12}/_{36}$
    b. $^1/_{36}$ e. $^7/_9$
    c. $^2/_6$

CHAPTER 2

Significant figures and scientific notation

In our work we will often be concerned with very large and very small quantities. Their conventional representation, whether by whole numbers, fractions, or decimals, have certain inadequacies in both form and accuracy that we will deal with in this chapter.

ACCURACY OF NUMBERS. The *accuracy* with which a quantity is represented should be consistent with the accuracy used in determining it. Although we employ approximate values for measured or computed quantities in virtually all practical calculations, we want to make sure not to lose needed accuracy and not to carry out unnecessarily accurate measurements or computations. Nor must we mislead anyone into assuming much more or much less accuracy than is actually present.

Measurement with a continuous scale. When a number of items is counted—the number of films taken today, the number of treatment fields on Mr. Brown, the number of vials of technetium (^{99m}Tc) received this morning, etc.—the answer should be *exact* and *precise*. Any deviation from the proper result is a definite *mistake*. However, when we measure a quantity that is continuous, such as length, mass, or time, the situation is completely different. Measuring the length of a rectangle against a centimeter scale is illustrated in Fig. 2-1. At a quick glance the rectangle appears to have a length of about 4 cm. Reading the scale to the nearest millimeter, we can see that the rectangle is about 4.2 cm long. Looking closer, we can locate the end of the rectangle about $^7/_{10}$ of the way from 4.1 to 4.2, which makes the length about 4.17 cm. Greater accuracy is not possible with this scale.

One might think that the precise length of a rectangle could be obtained if, instead of the simple scale illustrated we used a *vernier caliper* or, even better, a *micrometer*. Such refinements will yield a more accurate result, but the "true" precise length of the rectangle can never be defined or measured. In other words, greater care and improved tools and techniques can indeed produce higher accuracy, but not "absolute" precision. Aiming for an accuracy substantially better than required by the problem at hand is an expensive and unneccessary luxury. Assume, for example, that a shielding plan calls for 2 mm of lead on a wall. An extra 10% of lead would probably not overstrain the building and would obviously not lower the shielding capacity. If, on the other hand, a machine part is to fit tightly in a hole, it must be machined to high accuracy; if it is too large it will not fit and if it is too small it will be loose. A

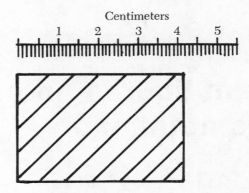

Fig. 2-1. Measurement of a length. Depending on the accuracy required, the length of the rectangle might be stated as 4 cm, 4.2 cm, or 4.17 cm.

10% margin in either direction would certainly not be acceptable accuracy in this case.

Let us return to Fig. 2-1. When we say the rectangle is 4 cm long, we mean that its length is closer to 4 cm than to 3 or 5 cm. One way to express this is by saying that the length (l) is greater than 3.5 cm and smaller than 4.5 cm. This can be written as $3.5 < l < 4.5$ cm or $l = 4.0 \pm 0.5$ cm. Similarly, when we say that the rectangle is 4.2 cm long, we imply that this more accurate measurement is 4.2 ± 0.05 cm. Finally, the value 4.17 cm could also be expressed as 4.17 ± 0.005 cm.

The value following the "plus or minus" sign is called the *error* or *uncertainty* in the number given. This is not an error in the sense of a mistake; it is an expression of the accuracy with which the number is measured or represented.

> **Example 2-1.** A patient is weighed to the nearest pound as 143 pounds. What is the uncertainty in this measure? The uncertainty is half of the smallest unit considered, here $\frac{1}{2}$ pound. The patient's weight might be written as 143 ± 0.5 pound.

> **Example 2-2.** If the field size of a beam is stated as $12 \times 17\frac{1}{2}$ cm, what is the error or uncertainty implied in these measures? Since one of the dimensions is given to the nearest half centimeter, it can be assumed that the uncertainty is not more than one half of this quantity, or $\frac{1}{4}$ centimeter.

Extremely large numbers and varying quantities. In some cases, there is in fact a precise numerical value, but the determination of the precise number would serve no purpose. For example, a standard lead brick contains about 30,000,000,000,000,000,000,000,000 lead (Pb) atoms. The precise number is immaterial to the shielding or mechanical properties of the brick, and a few billion billion atoms more or less would be extremely difficult to count. In such cases a manageable approximation of the number is better than the "exact" value.

Another case of approximation applies to numbers that may be precise in a specified instance but fluctuate with some parameter such as time. Take, for example, the number of occupied beds in a hospital. Except perhaps to the admitting clerk, the average number of occupied beds is probably more important than the exact number at a given instant, and sometimes the fluctuations are also important. Thus the figure 527 ± 32, as the average number of occupied beds over time, might be of more interest than 518, the number of occupied beds right now.

Precise numbers without exact fractional or decimal representations. Examples of precise numbers are the numerical constants that appear in mathematical formulas: π, $\sqrt{2}$, e, and log 2 (the constants π, e, and log 2 will be discussed in later chapters). Unfortunately, most of them do not have an exact representation either as decimals or as common fractions. For example, π has neither a terminating nor a repeating decimal representation. Therefore its symbol appears only in formulas and its approximate value is used in calculations. Reasonable approximations such as $\pi \cong 3.14$ or $\pi \cong 22/7$ are adequate for most purposes. A more accurate but less practical representation is $\pi \cong$ 3.1415926535897932384626.

SIGNIFICANT FIGURES AND SIGNIFICANT DECIMAL PLACES

The precise representation of an approximate number should contain the statement of an explicit error. For example, in the expression 4.20 ± 0.07, 0.07 is the explicit error. Even then it must be specified whether the expression represents the maximum possible error or an average error. Precise work in basic research or with certain types of physical or engineering measurements often requires allowance for an explicit error. For our purposes, however, it is rarely necessary.

SIGNIFICANT FIGURES. A simpler procedure, which retains the essence of the applicable error, is the method of counting *significant figures*. The *accuracy* of a number, or the magnitude of the implied error, is determined by the number of significant figures. By that we mean the number of digits used to express a value, excluding the zeros that merely locate the decimal point. For instance, the measurements of our rectangle, mentioned in the previous section, as 4 or 4.2 or 4.17 cm contain one, two, or three significant figures.

Rule 2-1. *Where there are no leading or trailing zeros, the number of digits is equal to the number of significant figures.*

> **Example 2-3.** How many significant figures are there in 320.45? Since there are no leading or trailing zeros, the number of significant figures is five.

What do we mean by a significant figure? A number correctly representing a quantity is assumed to be approximately accurate to one half the positional value of the last significant digit shown. Thus 527 is accurate to ±0.5 and $0.06 is accurate to $0.005 (half a cent or 5 mils). Beware of going too far in expressing accuracy. Assume, for example, that we measure with a rule the thickness of a piece of metal as about 3/64 of an inch, the decimal equivalent of which is 0.046875. If we now expressed this thickness as 0.046875, with the terminal 5 significant, we would imply an accuracy to ±0.0000005 inch—an absurd value for a measurement with a ruler, where accuracies better than ±0.005 inch are unlikely. The accepted convention is to designate the last significant digit by dropping all the trailing nonsignificant digits. The appropriate method for dropping nonsignificant digits will be described in a subsequent section of this chapter. The most basic guidelines for deciding which figures are significant are the position and purpose of zeros and decimal places in a given number.

Leading and trailing zeros. Consider a length measurement of 7 cm (one significant figure). This could also be expressed in other units, such as 0.07 m or 0.00007 km. Notice that the leading zeros are needed only to correctly place the decimal point and that changing the position of the decimal point does not change the number of significant figures.

Rule 2-2. *Leading zeros are not significant.*

Measurements in centimeters can also be expressed in millimeters. For example, 4.2 cm is the same as 42 mm. Both numbers have the same accuracy as expressed by their two significant figures. What happens if we write 7 cm as 70 mm? Does this imply two significant figures or greater accuracy than the original number? There are two methods to avoid this dilemma; one is to use scientific notation (explained in a subsequent section of this chapter), and the other method is to express the number with an explicit error as 70 ± 5 mm. It is incorrect to express it simply as 70 mm.

Rule 2-3. *Trailing zeros should only be retained if they are significant.*

This rule is often overlooked, however. When an estimate states that a certain construction project will cost ten million dollars, there is no indication of the number of significant figures employed. The context will occasionally clarify this somewhat. If, for example, the estimate suggests possible cost overruns of several millions, a reasonable conclusion would be that we deal with one significant figure.

Trailing zeros to the right of the decimal point are no problem. If they are nonsignificant, they can be discarded. If they are retained, they should be considered significant. Thus 20.0 has three significant figures.

Significant decimal places. Sometimes we talk of *significant decimal places* to the right (occasionally to the left) of the decimal point. Thus 7 cm has no significant decimal places, 0.07 mm has two and 0.00007 km has five. *Although shifting the decimal point to the left does not change the number of significant figures, it does change the number of significant decimal places.* The accuracy implied by the significant decimal places is the magnitude of the error (0.05 for 2.5) independent of the size of the quantity itself. Thus 6.02, 5063.61, and 0.03 all have two significant decimal places.

ROUNDING OFF. A frequent problem in mathematical computations is the need to eliminate digits that are not significant. For example, if we calculate 5% sales tax on 27¢, we obtain 1.35¢, not a practical amount of money. In normal usage, nothing smaller than one cent (or even one dollar in some cases) is considered significant. If a number includes some nonsignificant digits, they must be removed to avoid implying an unwarranted accuracy.

A similar situation is the approximate representation of nonrepeating decimals (such as π or $\sqrt{2}$). Earlier we represented the value of π with 23 significant figures (several thousand are known). This representation is much more accurate than necessary for such ordinary uses as the circumference, area, and volume problems that will be discussed in Chapter 4. It is often practical to eliminate digits that will not materially affect the numerical result we are seeking, even though they are theoretically significant. The correct process of removing nonsignificant digits is called *rounding off.*

Mechanics of rounding off. In rounding off, certain trailing digits are eliminated. What is the effect on the remaining digits? Usually only the rightmost (least significant) digit retained is affected. Rounding off is the reverse of the process discussed earlier in this chapter. That is, we take a number and express it in *less* accurate terms. For example, 4.17, with three significant digits and two significant decimal places, could be rounded off to two significant figures or one significant decimal place and expressed as 4.2. In this case we have represented our number by a less accurate one. In doing this we choose the closest value of the lower accuracy; 4.2 is closer to 4.17 than 4.1.

What are the mechanics of rounding off? In dropping a single digit, we have two choices. If the digit to be dropped is 6, 7, 8, or 9, we increase the last retained digit by one. This was the situation when 4.17 was rounded off to 4.2. If the digit to be dropped is 4, 3, 2, 1, or 0, we do not increase the last retained digit. For example, if we round 4.2 to the nearest digit, the result is 4.

> **Example 2-4.** Round 5.73 to two figures. Since we are dropping a 3, the last digit retained is unchanged. The rounded result is 5.7.

If the digit to be dropped is a 5, the situation is not so simple. Where we know that the value is actually slightly less than 5, say 4.95, we would round "down" and not change the last digit retained. If it is slightly greater, say 5.13, then we round up. For example, rounding 51.4503 and 8.6497 to one decimal place gives 51.5 and 8.6.

Because of the problems involved in rounding 5, it is best to round off all digits to be dropped at once rather than one at a time. For example, if we had rounded 8.6497 one digit at a time, we would have obtained 8.650 and then 8.65. This last gives the appearance of an exact 5, with the questions that go with rounding it off. Yet if we round all three right-hand digits at once it is obvious that rounded to one decimal place the proper expression is 8.6 and not 8.7.

> **Example 2-5.** Round 52.7551 to four significant figures. Because the

trailing digits to be dropped are 51, we will round up. Thus the result of the rounding is 52.76.

Another method of dealing with the problem of a 5 is to round up if that makes the retained digit even and not to round up if the retained decimal is already even. That is, 1.5, 2.5, and 3.5 would round to 2, 2, and 4, respectively. The logic behind this rule is that it tends to preserve the average in a large group of numbers.

Applications of rounding off. Sometimes the nature of our problem dictates whether we will round up or round down. This is not only restricted to rounding the digit 5. For example, suppose we have calculated that a certain situation required 0.7 inches of shielding by lead bricks 2 inches thick. The 0.7 inches is 0.35 (or less than one half) of one brick. If we rounded this to the nearest brick, the result would be 0, or no brick and no shielding! Such a result is plainly unacceptable; it is much better to overshield with one brick than to undershield with none. In a shielding problem we will almost always round up unless the amount being rounded is insignificant. If we had calculated 2.01 inches of lead, 2 inches would undoubtedly be acceptable. Similarly, if we need a rod that must pass through a hole with a 3.7 cm diameter, and rods come in whole centimeters only, we obtain a rod 3 cm thick and not 4 cm thick. These examples show that the practical nature of the quantity under consideration may tell us which way to round off. We must ask ourselves if there would be any problem should the result be slightly larger or slightly smaller than exact and then act accordingly.

A procedure called *conservative calculation* is used to ascertain the maximum or the minimum that a quantity can safely reach. This is especially important in radiation protection studies. Our decision about whether to round up or down here will depend on the result that it will have on the final value.

> **Example 2-6.** In personnel exposure records, 10 mrem or 0.01 rem (rem is the abbreviation for "roentgen-equivalent man") or less is considered insignificant. Supposing we wish to round our annual totals of exposures received to the nearest 0.1 rem, how do we round 3.640 rem and 1.605 rem? The number 3.640 is significantly greater than 3.600 (it is greater than 3.61); we should round it up to 3.7 rem. However, 1.605 is not significantly greater than 1.600. In fact, it is far less than 1.61 and can be rounded down to 1.6.

> **Example 2-7.** The safe maximum for a radionuclide storage container has been calculated. We wish to express the result to the nearest 100 millicuries (mCi). Should we round the calculated result up or down? If we round up in this case, we may exceed the safe limit for the container. We must round our result down.

SIGNIFICANT FIGURES IN CALCULATIONS. When mathematical operations use only precise quantities, the results should be exact. However, when approximate numbers are included, the result is necessarily approximate. Although we normally wish to be as accurate as possible in a calculation, the result should not be expressed to greater accuracy than is provided by the available data.

Addition and subtraction. Suppose we want to add 1.2 and 3.74. These numbers have one and two significant decimal places and two and three significant figures, respectively. They add to 4.94 if we disregard the implied uncertainties. The minimum values that these quantities can have are 1.15 and 3.735. For those the sum is at least 4.885. Similarly, their maximum possible values are 1.25 and 3.745, with a sum of 4.995. This addition can also be expressed with explicit errors as $(1.2 \pm 0.05) + (3.74 \pm 0.005) = 4.94 \pm 0.055$. The explicit errors can be added separately. The largest share of the explicit error (0.05 out of 0.055) is contributed by the 1.2, which is least accurate with respect to the number of significant decimal places. Thus most of the uncertainty, which at best is only a crude estimate, is contributed by this source. If we neglect the smaller contribution to the uncertainty, then the overall uncertainty is $\pm$ 0.05. Hence the answer should be expressed with one significant decimal place, as 4.9. Unless we choose to write explicit errors, this is the proper representation of our sum. By the same token, 4.94 is not a proper representation because it implies an accuracy that does not exist.

This example illustrates that the uncertainty in an addition operation is adequately approximated by the uncertainty in the less accurate quantity in the expression, that is, the number with the fewest significant decimal places. Because the uncertainty in the result is approximately equal to the uncertainty in the least accurate quantity in the expression, the number of significant decimal places in the correctly represented result is equal to the number of significant decimal places in the less accurate term. This rule also applies to the addition of more than two terms and to subtractions. It can be expressed as follows:

Rule 2-4. *For a sum or difference the number of significant decimal places in the result is equal to the number of significant decimal places in the term with the least number of significant decimal places.*

> **Example 2-8.** How do you write the answer for the subtraction 20. − 2.00? The first quantity has no significant decimal places, so the result should also have no places. The result is 18 (not 18.0 or 18.00).

Multiplication and division. Suppose we want to multiply a given number with an explicit error, say $35.4 \pm .05$, by a precise number, say 10. The result is 354 ± 0.5. Notice that both the number and the error are scaled by the multiplication. The relative error, that is, the ratio of the error to the number itself, remains the same. In our example the relative error is $\dfrac{0.05}{35.4} = \dfrac{0.5}{354} \cong$

0.0014. We see that multiplication of a nonprecise number by an exact number does not change the relative accuracy with which the nonprecise number is known. The same can be shown to be true for division.

A number written with a certain number of *significant figures* has an implied relative error or, in other words, the relative error is determined essentially by the number of significant figures. Thus multiplication or division of a nonprecise number by a precise number should not change the number of significant figures.

Example 2-9. The formula for the circumference (distance around) of a circle is πd, where d is the diameter of the circle. What is the correct representation of the circumference of a circle with a diameter of 2.4 cm? The quantity π is a precise quantity; however, as will be discussed in a later section, we are justified in using a three-figure approximation: 3.14. If we simply carry out the multiplication, the result is 7.536. However, we must represent our answer with only two significant figures, since 2.4 has only two figures. The correct representation for the circumference is 7.5 cm. Note that 8, 7.54, and 7.536 cm are all incorrect representations because they imply either too much or too little accuracy.

If two numbers, both with explicit errors, are multiplied or divided, the accuracy of the result is determined completely by the less accurate of the two quantities involved. This is expressed in the following rule:

Rule 2-5. *For a product or quotient, the number of significant figures in the result is equal to that of the term with fewer significant figures.*

Example 2-10. What is the correct form for the result of the multiplication of 20 by 0.2? Since the second term has only one significant figure, the result must have only one. The result is correctly expressed as 4 or 4., not 4.0 or 4.00.

When several mathematical operations are performed, rule 2-4 (for addition and subtraction) or rule 2-5 (for multiplication and division) can be applied at every step. In multistep operations it is customary to carry *one* nonsignificant digit through all intermediate steps and to round it off as the very last step. If this is not done, excessive errors may be generated by rounding off. On the other hand, if several nonsignificant digits are carried through the calculation, unnecessary work will have to be performed. In working with a computer or calculator, there is usually no rounding during calculation unless the number of columns available in the machine is exceeded. Rounding off at the end of the calculation is particularly important here and must be done by human judgment in almost all systems.

Acceptable accuracy of computational factors. When we carry out operations with mathematical quantities, we must not represent the various factors with too much or too little accuracy. If we use too much, it may take excessive time and effort to obtain or express the result. If we use too little, the result may be unacceptable.

How much accuracy should we use? We can represent π to as many significant decimal places as we wish, or measure a length to a few thousandths of an inch. Is it worth it? Usually there are clues either in the other data supplied or in the nature of the answer sought.

As we said before, it is acceptable to carry one nonsignificant digit throughout the calculation. If we then want to add to a value expressed to two significant decimal places another quantity, it is adequately represented to three significant decimal places. Similarly, for multiplication or division, one significant figure more than in the least accurate factor or in the result is adequate.

> **Example 2-11.** The length of the block in Figure 2-1 is to be added to the width to determine the perimeter. The width is known to be 3.2 cm; what length should be used? Because the width has one significant decimal place, the length should have two significant places. The value 4.17 cm should be used.

> **Example 2-12.** For the same block as in the previous example, the width is to be multiplied by the length to determine the area. The width has two significant figures, so the length should have three. Again, 4.17 cm should be used.

> **Example 2-13.** A length is to be multiplied by $\sqrt{2}$. If the length is 35.6 cm, what representation should be used for $\sqrt{2}$ ($\sqrt{2} = 1.4142136\ldots$)? Since the length is given to three significant figures, $\sqrt{2}$ should be represented to four figures: $\sqrt{2} = 1.414$.

SCIENTIFIC NOTATION

Numerical representation of certain quantities may be impractical with ordinary decimals. For example, it is inconvenient to write very small numbers, such as the charge on an electron, 0.00000000000000000016 coulomb, as a simple decimal even though there is nothing incorrect in this expression. This holds just as true with very large numbers. For example, a curie can be defined as an activity comprising 37,000,000,000 disintegrations each second. Since this number is exact, the nine zeros are significant. However, for a large, experimentally evaluated number, the zeros are a real problem. Thus if we write the speed of light as 300,000,000 m/second, we also imply the accuracy, although in this case the expression is accurate to only three figures. But there is no way of telling this from the way it is written.

Scientific notation allows a representation of very large or very small quantities without the large number of leading or trailing zeros. This is particularly important for calculators or other representations in which the number of digits available is restricted. When we use scientific notation in manual calculations, we can express, by the number of significant figures, both the quantity and the accuracy.

STANDARD REPRESENTATION. Scientific notation makes use of powers of 10. The exponential notation and its significance are discussed in greater detail in Chapter 7. Suffice it to note here that, for example,

$$10^3 = \underbrace{10 \times 10 \times 10}_{3 \text{ tens}} = \underbrace{1{,}000}_{3 \text{ zeros}}$$

or in general:

$$10^n = \underbrace{10 \times 10 \times \ldots \times 10 \times 10}_{n \text{ tens}} = \underbrace{100 \ldots 00.}_{n \text{ zeros}} \qquad \text{Formula 2-1}$$

For negative powers of 10, such as 10^{-2}, the product 10's appear in the denominator: $10^{-2} = \dfrac{1}{\underbrace{10 \times 10}_{2 \text{ tens}}} = 0.\underbrace{01}_{2 - 1 \text{ zeros}}.$

In general, for negative powers:

$$10^{-n} = \dfrac{1}{\underbrace{10 \times 10 \times \ldots \times 10 \times 10}_{n \text{ tens}}} = 0.\underbrace{00 \ldots 01}_{n - 1 \text{ zeros}} \qquad \text{Formula 2-2}$$

In the boxed material, some powers of 10 and their common decimal representations are shown. Note particularly 10^1 and 10^0.

POWERS OF TEN

$10^4 = 10{,}000$		$10^0\ \ = 1$
$10^3 = 1{,}000$		$10^{-1} = 0.1$
$10^2 = 100$		$10^{-2} = 0.01$
$10^1 = 10$		$10^{-3} = 0.001$

There are many ways we can express a quantity as the product of a number and a power of 10. For example, 300 can be written as 300×10^0, 30.0×10^1, 3.0×10^2, 0.3×10^3, 0.03×10^4, $3{,}000 \times 10^{-1}$, and so forth. Out of these possibilities it is conventional in handwritten material to use the form in which there is one digit to the left of the decimal point. Thus the conventional representation for 300 in scientific notation is 3.00×10^2. This is the most generally accepted form, but others are used and they provide, of course, the same information.

In the conventional form of scientific notation, all digits except the first come after the decimal. Accordingly, all nonsignificant digits can be dropped. For example, if the 300 just mentioned is accurate only to the nearest hundred, then there is only one significant figure and the correct representation is $3. \times 10^2$. If the 300 is accurate to five significant figures (to the nearest $1/100$ of a unit), the correct representation is 3.0000×10^2.

> **Example 2-14.** Write eleven million (11,000,000) in scientific notation; assume three significant figures. Since three significant figures will be used, the first portion of the number is 1.10. The appropriate power of 10 is 7. Thus the desired representation is 1.10×10^7.

How can we routinely translate numbers in ordinary representation to scientific notation? We can think of the process as consisting of two parts. The first part involves moving the decimal point to the appropriate position and the second is to multiply by the appropriate power of 10. If we move the decimal point one position to the left, we effectively divide by 10, that is, 423.65 divided by 10 is 42.365. If we wish to move the decimal point one position to the left but retain the overall value, we must multiply our number by 10 (or 10^1); $423.65 = 42.365 \times 10$. If the decimal point is moved two positions to the left, the appropriate factor of 10 is 10^2; $423.65 = 4.2365 \times 10^2$. Three positions to the left will require a factor of 10^3, and so on.

> **Example 2-15.** Represent 365.24 in scientific notation. We move the decimal point two places to the left and multiply by 10^2: 3.6524×10^2.

When the decimal point is moved one position to the right, a number is effectively multiplied by 10. If we wish to do this but retain the overall value, we must divide our new number by 10. Division by 10 is equivalent to multiplication by $1/10$ or by 10^{-1}; $423.65 = 4236.5 \times 10^{-1}$. If we move the decimal point two places to the right, we must multiply by 10^{-2}. Three places to the right will call for multiplication by 10^{-3}, and so on.

> **Example 2-16.** Write 0.0043 in scientific notation. Here we shift the decimal point three places to the right and multiply by 10^{-3} to compensate. The result is 4.3×10^{-3}.

The reverse process, going from scientific notation to common notation, is carried out in essentially the same way, and the power of 10 tells us how to move the decimal point. For example, to write 4.73×10^2 without the power of 10 requires that the decimal point be moved two places to the right.

Similarly, if the power of 10 is negative, the decimal point must be moved the appropriate number of positions to the left.

> **Example 2-17.** Write 3.4×10^{-4} in regular notation. The 10^{-4} requires the shifting of the decimal point four places to the left. To be able to do this, we must generate sufficient leading zeros. Thus $3.4 \times 10^{-4} = 0.00034$.

> **Example 2-18.** Write 4.7×10^5 in regular notation. The 10^5 requires that the decimal point be moved five places to the right. Nonsignificant trailing zeros must be added. Thus $4.7 \times 10^5 = 470,000$.

Scientific notation is a convenient representation of large and small numbers. It also permits us to use exactly the appropriate number of significant figures. For these two reasons, it is often used in scientific and engineering applications.

ALTERNATE REPRESENTATIONS. A variation from the customary representation places the decimal point one column to the left of the position in the conventional scientific notation. The first character encountered in this form is either a zero or the decimal point itself. Thus 27 is written as 0.27×10^2 or $.27 \times 10^2$ instead of 2.7×10^1. Here the power of 10 is one greater than in the conventional representation.

Other common variants are mostly associated with the representation of the power of 10. One of them uses a letter, most frequently E or D. Thus whereas three million in the conventional representation with three significant figures is 3.00×10^6, in the "E" representation it could be $3.00E6$. Note that the E can be read as "times 10 to the . . ." The D form is exactly the same as the E form. Sometimes, particularly on calculators, the E or D is dropped and only a gap appears so that 3.00×10^6 appears as $3.00\ 6$. The power of 10 is often represented as a two- or three-digit number with leading zeros, if necessary, as in $3.00\ 006$ or $3.00\ D06$. Usually, if the power is positive, there is no sign for it, but this is not always true; another representation of three million is $3.00E\ +06$. Negative powers are always indicated by the minus sign. Note that in this notation $5.4\ -02$ does not mean 3.4, but rather 0.054.

OPERATIONS IN SCIENTIFIC NOTATION. Major advantages of scientific notation are its compactness and the unambiguous way in which it indicates the degree of accuracy by the number of significant figures. However, arithmetical operations in scientific notation require special attention when it comes to handling the powers of 10.

Addition and subtraction. Normally, in adding or subtracting decimal numbers, lining up the decimal point is adequate. In scientific notation the problem is more involved.

One way to avoid mistakes is to convert the quantities to be added or subtracted to regular form. These can then be added or subtracted in the normal way, and the answer converted back to scientific notation.

> **Example 2-19.** Add 3.7×10^3 and 2.11×10^2. First, convert these to the regular forms 3,700 and 211. These add to make 3,911. Notice that the trailing 11 is not significant, since the trailing zeros in 3,700 are not significant. The scientific notation form is 3.9×10^3.

> **Example 2-20.** Subtract 2.6×10^{-8} from 3.64×10^{-7}. Converting these to the usual decimal form we obtain:

$$\begin{array}{r} 0.000000364 \\ -0.000000026 \\ \hline 0.000000338 \end{array}$$

Because each number defining the differences had nine significant decimal places, the result also has nine, that is, the final 8 is significant. In scientific notation the result is 3.38×10^{-7}.

This method of converting from scientific notation and then back is recommended for the average user of this text. However, for the more adventurous there is another way that is both faster and more dangerous. If the powers of 10 are the same, the numbers can be added or subtracted directly. The power of 10 for the result is the same as the power for the two terms in the sum or difference. This is a consequence of the distributive law. For example, the addition of 3.41×10^4 and 4.6×10^4 can be written as (3.41×10^4) + (4.6×10^4). Because 10^4 is common to both terms, it can be factored out as ($3.41 + 4.6$) $\times 10^4$. Then the addition becomes easy and the result is 8.0×10^4 (the nonsignificant trailing 1 has been dropped). If the powers of 10 are not the same, they can be brought into agreement by adjusting the decimal points.

Multiplication and division. Multiplication and division in scientific notation are simpler than addition and subtraction.

Multiplication is carried out through regrouping. For example, (2.0×10^3) $\times$ (4.6×10^1) is equal to (2.0×4.6) $\times$ ($10^3 \times 10^1$). The first pair of parentheses contains a normal multiplication, 2.0×4.6, which is readily carried out, resulting in 9.2 (only two significant figures retained). The second term is a multiplication of two powers, discussed in detail in Chapter 7. Suffice to say here that $10^3 \times 10^1 = 10^4$ in particular, and $10^n \times 10^m = 10^{n+m}$ in general. Multiplication in scientific notation can be represented by this formula:

$$\boxed{(a \times 10^n) \times (b \times 10^m) = (a \times b) \times 10^{n+m}} \qquad \text{Formula 2-3}$$

This formula makes multiplication of very large or very small numbers quite easy.

Example 2-21. Multiply 5.1×10^5 by 1.6×10^{-19}. Applying the formula, this product can be written as $(5.1 \times 1.6) \times 10^{5-19} = 8.16 \times 10^{-14}$. Since the terms were given to two significant figures, this result should be rounded off to 8.2×10^{-14}.

Example 2-22. Find $(3.0 \times 10^8)^2$. This can be considered as $(3.0 \times 10^8) \times (3.0 \times 10^8) = (3.0 \times 3.0) \times 10^{8+8} = 9.0 \times 10^{16}$.

A similar approach can be taken for division. The formula equivalent to $2 - 3$ can be shown as follows:

$$(a \times 10^n) \div (b \times 10^m) = (a \div b) \times 10^{n-m} \qquad \text{Formula 2-4}$$

Example 2-23. Find $(4.4 \times 10^5) \div (3.1 \times 10^2)$. This is $(4.4 \div 3.1) \times 10^{5-2} = 1.4 \times 10^3$. Here only two significant figures are retained.

Example 2-24. Find the inverse of 1.6×10^{-19}. The inverse of a number is equal to 1 divided by the number. In scientific notation, 1 is 1.00×10^0. (The two zeros were added to give adequate accuracy.) Thus the inverse is $1.00 \times 10^0 \div 1.6 \times 10^{-19} = (1.00 \div 1.6) \times 10^{0-(-19)} = 0.63 \times 10^{19}$, or 6.3×10^{18}.

Powers and roots. Scientific notation facilitates the computation of powers and roots. Example 2-22 showed the way to compute a power. In general terms:

$$(a \times 10^n)^k = (a^k) \times 10^{kn} \qquad \text{Formula 2-5}$$

Example 2-25. Find $(1.6 \times 10^{-19})^4$. According to formula 2-5, this is $(1.6)^4 \times 10^{4(-19)} = 6.6 \times 10^{-76}$.

As will be discussed in detail in Chapter 7, the mth root of a number is equivalent to the $\frac{1}{m}$-th power, that is, $\sqrt[m]{x} = x^{1/m}$. Thus a formula for roots can be derived from formula 2-5:

$$\sqrt[m]{(a \times 10^n)} = (a \times 10^n)^{1/m} = \sqrt[m]{a} \times 10^{n/m} \qquad \text{Formula 2-6}$$

Example 2-26. Find the square root of 9.0×10^{-4}. This is equal to $\sqrt{9.0} \times 10^{-4/2} = 3.0 \times 10^{-2}$.

This example can be worked out easily because the number is an exact square and the power of 10 is even. In general, it is easiest to force the power of 10 in formula 2-6 to be exactly divisible by the root m. For example, the square root of 1.6×10^{-19} is most readily taken by changing it to 16×10^{-20}, or 0.16×10^{-18}. If this is not done $10^{n/m}$ will result in a fractional power (or root) of 10. This adjustment of the power of 10 is always possible; the root of the decimal number may require the use of tables or a calculator.

> **Example 2-27.** Find the cube root of 1.6×10^{-19}. Since this involves a cube root, adjust the power of 10 so that it will be divisible by 3. The form 0.16×10^{-18} is suitable. The cube root of this is $\sqrt[3]{0.16} \times 10^{-18/3} \cong 0.54 \times 10^{-6}$. In this case the power of 10 is easily handled, but $\sqrt[3]{0.16}$ cannot be found so simply.

CHAPTER REVIEW

1. Can all quantities be evaluated to high accuracy? Why?
2. Is it always desirable to represent quantities with as much accuracy as is available?
3. What is a significant figure?
4. How are significant figures related to accuracy?
5. Are leading zeros significant?
6. When are trailing zeros significant?
7. In ordinary numbers, can we always determine which digits are significant?
8. How do significant decimal places differ from significant figures?
9. Which nonsignificant digits normally cause us to round up? Round down?
10. Why, in certain cases, do we only round figures up?
11. Are significant figures or significant decimal places the important measure of accuracy in addition and subtraction?
12. In multiplication and division, which is important for accuracy—significant figures or significant decimal places?
13. How many figures or decimal places should be used in a computation?
14. How many figures or decimal places should be used in the approximate representation of an exact number?
15. What is scientific notation?
16. Why is scientific notation handy?
17. How do we add in scientific notation?
18. How do we know the accuracy of a number in scientific notation?
19. How do we multiply in scientific notation?

PROBLEMS
Problems paralleling chapter examples

1. (2-1) In radiotherapy the dose given for a certain treatment is either 5,000 rads or 5,500 rads, depending on the condition of the patient. What are the uncertainties implied in these numbers?
2. (2-2) The usual dosage for a certain scan procedure is 4 mCi. What is the uncertainty implied by this prescription?
3. (2-3) How many significant figures are there in the number 27.4?
4. (2-4) Round off 4.263 to three figures.
5. (2-5) Round off 5.347 to two figures.
6. (2-6) A protection calculation accurate to 0.1 mm calls for 2.55 mm. If lead is available in 2.0, 2.5 and 3.0 mm thicknesses, which thickness should we use?
7. (2-7) A molybdenum-technetium cow will yield 183 mCi of technetium at a certain time. If an institution uses technetium for radiopharmaceutical preparations in units of 50 mCi, should this number be rounded up to 200 mCi or down to 150 mCi?

8. **(2-8)** What is the correct representation of the sum $45.3 + 2$?

9. **(2-9)** What is the correct representation of the result of $2.72 \div 3.0$?

10. **(2-11)** The area of a floor is to be calculated to two significant figures. How many significant figures should we obtain in measuring the length and the width?

11. **(2-12)** The activity 10.1 mCi is to be multiplied by hand with a decay value obtained from a table. The tabulated value is 0.9773466. What value should be used in the product?

12. **(2-14)** Write 1,600 years in scientific notation, assuming two significant figures.

13. **(2-15)** Write 30 years in conventional scientific notation.

14. **(2-16)** Write 0.025 in conventional scientific notation.

15. **(2-17)** Write 2.752×10^{-2} without using a power of 10, that is, write the number in the ordinary decimal notation.

16. **(2-18)** Write the exact number 3.6×10^3 without using scientific notation.

17. **(2-19)** Add 3.4×10^3 and 2.71×10^5. Express the result in scientific notation with the proper number of significant figures.

18. **(2-20)** Subtract 8.6×10^{-3} from 7.9×10^{-4}. Express the result in scientific notation.

19. **(2-21)** Multiply 1.6×10^{-19} by 6.023×10^{26}.

20. **(2-22)** Express $(1.6 \times 10^{-19})^2$ as a single number in scientific notation.

21. **(2-23)** Calculate $(1.24 \times 10^1) \div (6.6 \times 10^2)$.

22. **(2-24)** Find the inverse of 3×10^8.

23. **(2-25)** Find the cube of 4.8×10^{-10}.

24. **(2-26)** Find the square root of 1.21×10^6. Note that $\sqrt{1.21} = 1.1$.

25. **(2-27)** Find the square root of 4.9×10^7.

Problems related to this chapter

26. For the numbers below give the number of significant figures.
    a. 54.6
    b. 0.002
    c. −1.473
    d. \$0.64
    e. 12.4

27. For the numbers below give the number of significant decimal places.
    a. 32¢
    b. \$0.27
    c. 660
    d. 1.25
    e. 6

28. Without calculating the following expressions, give for each the number of significant figures in the result.
    a. $16.0 \div 2.1$
    b. $17 \div 3$
    c. $12 \div 6.0$
    d. 18×2
    e. 4.26×3.14

29. Without calculating the following expressions, give for each the number of significant decimal places in the result.
    a. $27.1 - 27.02$
    b. $18.6 + 186$
    c. $3.14 + 1.0$
    d. $22.60 - 1.3$
    e. $3 + 2$

30. The cube root of 2 is approximately 1.25992105. Round this value to the number of significant figures indicated.
    a. Six figures
    b. Four figures
    c. Three figures
    d. Two figures
    e. One figure

31. Round off each of the following numbers to two significant figures less than the number shown. Use scientific notation to represent any number that would otherwise require leading or trailing zeros.
    a. 1.456
    b. 27.31
    c. 526
    d. 0.0035
    e. −182

32. Express the following numbers in scientific notation.
    a. 2,576
    b. 22.55
    c. −4.8
    d. 0.0021
    e. 345.678

33. Express the following numbers without using scientific notation.
    a. 5.92×10^1
    b. 1.24×10^{-2}
    c. -4.5×10^{-1}

34. Calculate the following, expressing the answer as a single number in scientific notation.
    a. $(3.5 \times 10^6)^2$
    b. $(4.1 \times 10^{-2}) \times (8.8 \times 10^{-1})$
    c. $\sqrt{2.25 \times 10^{12}}$
    d. $(5.27 \times 10^2) \div (2.0 \times 10^4)$
    e. $(47.6 \times 10^5) \div (2.1 \times 10^{-5})$

35. In calculating the sum of the four numbers 47.3, 20.4, 5.6, and 0.02, should we neglect 0.02 by setting it to zero?

36. A room is a square, 3.2 m on a side. The diagonal of this square room can be shown, by the methods discussed in Chapter 4, to be $3.2 \times \sqrt{2}$. In calculating this value by hand, what approximate value of the $\sqrt{2}$ should we use? ($\sqrt{2} \cong 1.41421$).

37. The pythagorean theorem (Chapter 4) shows that the diagonal of a rectangle of sides l and w is $\sqrt{l^2 + w^2}$. If we calculate this diagonal for an object 2.7×1.2, using an electronic calculator, we obtain the length of the diagonal as 2.954657. Give the correct representation of this answer.

Objective questions

38. The number 2.01×10^{-3} is equal to:
    a. 0.00201
    b. 0.99
    c. 2.01
    d. -6.7
    e. -201

39. The number 2,571 rounded to two significant figures is properly written as:
    a. 2.571×10^3
    b. 25.71×10^2
    c. 26
    d. 2.6×10^3
    e. 25.7×10^2

40. The expression 5.0×10^{-1} is not equivalent to which of the following:
    a. -5
    b. $\frac{1}{2}$
    c. 50%
    d. 0.5

41. The expression $2.1 \times 10^3 \times 4.0 \times 10^{-2}$ is equal to:
    a. 8.4×10
    b. 8.4×10^{-6}
    c. 6.1×10
    d. -8.4×10^5
    e. -6.1×10^5

42. The expression $\sqrt{4 \times 10^6}$ is equal to:
    a. 2×10^6
    b. 2×10^3
    c. 4×10^3
    d. 3×10^2
    e. 12

43. The number of significant digits present in the result of a multiplication is determined by the number of significant _____ present in the _____ significant term.
    a. decimal places, least
    b. figures, least
    c. decimal places, most
    d. figures, most

44. The number of significant decimal places in the number 21.01 is:
    a. 1
    b. 2
    c. 3
    d. 4
    e. 5

45. There are three significant figures in a certain result obtained on a calculator. On the calculator this result appears as 10.563. The answer we should quote is:
    a. 10
    b. 10.6
    c. 10.56
    d. 10.563
    e. none of these

46. The correct representation of 21.10×2.0 is:
    a. 42
    b. 42.2
    c. 42.20
    d. 42.200

47. The sum of $6.3 \times 10^3 + 3.2 \times 10^3$ is:
    a. 3.1
    b. 9.5×10^3
    c. 9.5×10^6
    d. 9.5×10^9

48. The product of $(4.1 \times 10^2)\,(2.0 \times 10^3)$ is:
    a. 12.3×10^6
    b. 12.3×10^5
    c. 12.3×10^4
    d. 8.2×10^6
    e. 8.2×10^5

49. The number of significant figures in 3.75×10^4 is:
    a. 1
    b. 2
    c. 3
    d. 4
    e. 5

50. The sum of $4.2 \times 10^2 + 5.1 \times 10^1$ is:
    a. 5.52×10^3
    b. 4.7×10^2
    c. 4.71×10^2
    d. 9.3×10^2
    e. 9.3×10^3

51. The product of $(3.0 \times 10^4)^2$ is:
    a. 6.0×10^4
    b. 9.0×10^4
    c. 3.0×10^8
    d. 6.0×10^8
    e. 9.0×10^8

CHAPTER 3

Basic algebra

Algebra differs from arithmetic in that it uses letters to represent numbers. Letters are also used in mathematical formulas and, therefore, algebra is a key technique in deriving and modifying formulas.

Algebra uses the same operations as mathematics. It clarifies and deepens the meaning of these operations and makes them more generally applicable.

NOTATION AND EXPRESSIONS

In ordinary arithmetic, specific numerical values are manipulated and combined by mathematical operations. Thus 2 + 4 means that the quantity 2 and the quantity 4 are to be combined by the mathematical operation of addition. In algebra the quantities are not explicitly written down in numerical form, but rather are represented by suitable nonnumerical symbols, usually the letters of the alphabet. Thus simple addition might be expressed as "$a + b$."

REPRESENTATION OF NUMBERS BY LETTERS. We may know that a certain item has or will have a specific numerical value but not what that value is. For example, the area of the floor in x-ray room No. 1 is well-defined and can be measured, but we may not know its value at this moment. Similarly, the number of gamma cameras a hospital will own in six months, if not definite now, will be established in six months. If we have to manipulate such quantities, we often cannot afford to wait until their actual value is known. We might compromise by writing in words the entire definition "the number of patients sitting in waiting room B at 2 PM," but it is much more convenient to choose a letter or group of letters to represent this quantity. Thus "a" might represent the area of the floor in room No. 1 and "N" the number of patients. This is nothing but a set of abbreviations for numerical quantities. Besides both capital and lower case Roman letters, other symbols may be used as descriptors, such as Greek letters and subscripts (small letters set slightly below the others). For instance, the number of patients treated on Monday might be represented by N_M ("N sub M").

The symbols standing for numerical quantities are often called "unknowns," "variables," or "constants." There are slight differences between these terms: a *variable* implies that the quantity takes on different values in different situations; for example, the number of patients treated daily, or the number of technicians on vacation are quantities that change from day to day. An *unknown* is more likely to represent a definite number. In general, the first letters of the alphabet are used for unknowns and the last ones, particularly *x, y* and *z,* are used for variables. A *constant,* usually represented by *C* or *K,* is always an unchanging (but sometimes undefined) value.

ALGEBRAIC EXPRESSIONS. Once representations have been chosen for unknown quantities, they can be formally grouped together into an *algebraic expression.* For example, if the number of films taken in the morning is N_1 and the number of films taken in the afternoon is N_2, the total number of films for the day is "expressed" by $N_1 + N_2$.

> **Example 3-1.** Before a film is processed, a processor contains D_0 gm of developer. If a film uses *d* gm of developer, what is the expression for the amount of developer immediately after this processing? Because this represents a subtraction, the expression is $D_0 - d$.

Expressions consist of two or more numbers or variables joined by the appropriate mathematical operation. Thus $x + y$, $a \div b$, $\sqrt{c}$, $2b$, $W + 1$, and $\frac{1}{2}\pi r^2$ are all expressions. Note that the multiplication sign is usually omitted where there is no ambiguity, as in $2b$ and $\frac{1}{2}\pi r^2$.

A particularly simple and common expression is the addition of two variables, such as $a + b$, $p + q$, or $x + y$. This expression is known as a *binomial.* Some of the properties of binomials will be considered further in this chapter and in Chapter 9. An expression containing more than two terms may be called a *polynomial.*

Portions of an expression may be set off by parentheses. Thus $x + (a - 2)$ is the same as $x + a - 2$. The parentheses here, as in Chapter 1, determine the order of the operations and, in many cases, make for a more precise expression. In *arithmetic* the easiest method of solving expressions with parentheses consists of reducing the expression within a set of parentheses to a single number. In *algebra* this is usually not possible and the manipulation is more involved, as will be shown.

Because single algebraic variables stand for numbers, the expressions also represent numerical quantities. The associative, commutative, and distributive laws will hold for algebraic expressions in the same way as for numbers. Thus the commutative law of addition can be written as follows:

$$a + b = b + a$$

and of multiplication as:

$$xy = yx$$

The associative and distributive laws are particularly important for the correct manipulation of parentheses. The associative laws of addition and multiplication in algebra can be written as (the choice of symbols is arbitrary here):

$$C + (D + E) = (C + D) + E$$

and:

$$w(u \cdot v) = (w \cdot u)v$$

The distributive law can be written as follows:

$$x(y + z) = xy + xz$$

Formula 3-1

Notice that for the associative law parentheses are unimportant and can be dropped, as in $C + (D + E) = C + D + E$, without creating any ambiguity. The distributive law shows how an expression can be rewritten without parentheses.

> **Example 3-2.** Express $a(b - c)$ without parentheses. First, the expression can be changed to $a[b + (-c)]$. It is now in the form of formula 3-1, where $a = x$, $b = y$, and $(-c) = z$. Thus the expression can be written as $ab + a(-c)$. Because $a(-c) = -ac$, it can be written in final form without the parentheses as $ab - ac$.

When more than one operation is given in an expression, the order in which the operations are carried out follows the same rules in algebra as in arithmetic (Chapter 1). That is, powers or roots are performed first, then multiplication or division, and finally addition or subtraction. Parentheses can be used to modify this order.

In the case of numerical evaluations it is usually simplest to carry out the operations in the normally prescribed order. In arithmetic the result of each operation is a single number. In algebra this is usually not the case; in fact, the result of a mathematical operation involving two algebraic expressions is a new expression, which usually contains more terms than either of the original expressions. For example, the addition of the expressions $a + b$ and $b + c$ yields the expression $a + 2b + c$.

Possibly the simplest manipulation of an algebraic expression is its numerical evaluation. Here, numerical values are assigned to all unknowns, and all operations are actually carried out with numbers.

> **Example 3-3.** Evaluate the expression $2x + y$ when $x = 3$ and $y = -2$. Replacing x and y by their numerical values, we obtain the expression $2(3) + (-2) = 6 - 2 = 4$.

> **Example 3-4.** Evaluate the expression $A^2 + 3B$ when $A = 3$ and $B = 4$. This expression is equal to $3^2 + 3(4) = 9 + 12 = 21$.

> **Example 3-5.** Evaluate the expression $(x - 6)^2 - (x + 4)^2$ when $x = -2$. This becomes $(-2 - 6)^2 - (-2 + 4)^2 = (-8)^2 - (+2)^2 = 64 - 4 = 60$.

Even in those cases where numerical values are not known, expressions can still be manipulated primarily by means of the associative, commutative, and distributive laws. Also, we can add or subtract zero or multiply or divide by $+1$. These latter operations may not sound impressive, but in algebra, where 0 is equal to $x - x$ or $2a + b - (2a + b)$ and 1 is equal to $^y/_y$ or $(2a + b) \div (2a + b)$, they become powerful tools. These methods provide an unlimited number of ways to reorganize expressions. Only a few of these ways are of practical use. We will consider three ways to reorganize expressions: *collecting terms, ordering by power,* and *factoring.* Remember that these do not represent all manipulations possible, but only some of those that are useful. These manipulations are usually associated with the solution of equations, which is described in the section on equations later in this chapter.

Collecting terms is the grouping together of all terms containing the same variable—say x—and, if possible, simplifying their total.

> **Example 3-6.** Collect terms in the expression $6x + 2y + 4 - 3x -2y + 7$. Place all the "x" terms first, then the "y" terms, and finally the numerical terms to obtain $6x - 3x + 2y - 2y + 4 + 7$. This expression can be simplified to $3x + 11$.

> **Example 3-7.** Collect terms in the expression $x + 2y - 3z + 7 - ^1/_x + ^2/_y - ^3/_z$. This expression becomes $x - ^1/_x + 2y + ^2/_y - 3z - ^3/_z + 7$.

When terms contain two variables, they are usually grouped between the terms containing only one variable; $2xy$ would be between the "x" terms and the "y" terms; for example, $3x + 2xy - 5y$.

In *ordering by power,* the highest power is usually placed to the left and the lowest to the right.

> **Example 3-8.** Group $2x + 3x^2 - 4$ in order of power. The term x^2 has the highest power and 4 has the lowest. Thus the grouping is $3x^2 + 2x - 4$.

Expressions in which the highest power of a variable is one (as $3x + 2y$) are called *linear.* Those with the highest power of two (as $3x^2 + y$) are called *quadratic,* and those with the highest power of three, *cubic.* Notice that it is the term with the highest power that determines the power of the entire expression.

Factoring. A factor that is contained in all terms of an expression can be "factored out." In the expression $2ax + ay$ the term "a" is common to both. By reversing the distributive law (formula 3-1), we obtain:

$$a(2x) + a(y) = a(2x + y)$$

In the expression on the right, the term "a" is factored out.

> **Example 3-9.** Factor 2 from the expression $2x + 4y - 6z$. When 2 is removed from (divided into) each term, the results are x, $2y$ and $-3z$,

respectively. Thus the factored form of the expression is $2(x + 2y - 3z)$.

Example 3-10. Determine the common factor in the expression $2abx^2 + 10axyz$ and give the expression in factored form. It can be seen that 2, a, and x are all common factors; thus $2ax$ can be factored out. The factored form of the expression is then

$$2ax(bx + 5yz)$$

If there is a common factor for some but not all of the terms, the factoring can be carried out over the restricted group of terms. For example, $x^2 + 2x - 3$ can be factored by x for the first two terms as $x(x + 2) - 3$.

Factoring can also be used to simplify fractional expressions. A common factor in both numerator and denominator of a fraction can also be canceled out. For example, both the numerator and the denominator of $\dfrac{(bx + by)}{(2b^2 + bz)}$ have the common factor b. In factored form this expression becomes $\dfrac{b(x + y)}{b(2b + z)}$. The b can be canceled, yielding $\dfrac{x + y}{2b + z}$.

Example 3-11. Factor x out of the numerator and denominator of $\dfrac{x^2}{x^2 - x}$ and cancel. The numerator can be factored to yield $x(x)$; the denominator factors to $x(x - 1)$. After the factor x is canceled, the expression becomes $\dfrac{x}{(x - 1)}$.

Fractions are also added and subtracted in algebraic form. Just as in arithmetic, a common denominator must be found. A suitable denominator (although not necessarily the lowest) is obtained by multiplying the two denominators. As in arithmetic, the final fraction can often be simplified by factoring.

Example 3-12. Add $\dfrac{x}{y}$ and $\dfrac{x + 1}{y + 1}$. The common denominator is $y(y + 1)$ and the sum is $\dfrac{x(y + 1)}{y(y + 1)} + \dfrac{(x + 1)y}{y(y + 1)} = \dfrac{x(y + 1) + (x + 1)y}{y(y + 1)}$. If desired, the numerator can be written as $x(y + 1) + (x + 1)y = xy + x + xy + y = x + 2xy + y$.

Example 3-13. Express $\dfrac{1}{x + 1} - \dfrac{1}{x - 1}$ as a single fraction. This is equal to $\dfrac{x - 1}{(x + 1)(x - 1)} - \dfrac{x + 1}{(x + 1)(x - 1)}$

$$= \frac{x - 1 - x - 1}{(x + 1)(x - 1)} = \frac{-2}{(x + 1)(x - 1)} \, .$$

In some cases it may be desirable to add or delete parentheses. Parentheses are redundant when they do not change the value of an expression, as in $a + (b)$.

> **Example 3-14.** Are the parentheses in the expression $a \cdot (b \cdot c)$ redundant? Yes, because the value of the expression remains unchanged when the parentheses are removed.
>
> **Example 3-15.** Are the parentheses in the expression $c \cdot (a + b)$ redundant? No, because the expression $c \cdot a + b$ is not equal to the correct expression $c \cdot a + c \cdot b$ given by the distributive law.

When should we add or delete redundant parentheses? We should consider adding parentheses when it would lead to a more compact expression, as in the case of factoring just considered. Deleting parentheses is useful when a reorganization is possible. For example, the expression $a(b - c) + b(c - a) + c(a - b)$ can be expanded by using the distributive law to remove the parentheses: $ab - ac + bc - ab + ac - bc$. From the converted form we can see at a glance that the expression is equal to zero.

The distributive law is particularly useful in eliminating parentheses. Keep this in mind when dealing with negative signs outside parentheses or with binomials. In the expression $-(x + y - z)$, the minus sign before the parentheses is equivalent to a multiplication by -1. That means the expression equals $(-1) \cdot (x + y - z)$. The distributive law can now be used to produce the equivalent expression $(-1)x + (-1)y - (-1)z$, which is equal to $-x - y + z$. Comparison with the original form of the expression shows that the signs immediately in front of each term (note that the x had an implied $+$ in the initial expression) are all changed by the overall minus sign. For example $x - (y - z)$ is equal to $x - y + z$. Another important use of the distributive law is the treatment of polynomial products. The expression $(a + b)(c + d)$ can be considered for the application of the distributive law if $(a + b)$ is viewed as a single term. This law then yields the following:

$$(a + b)(c + d) = (a + b)c + (a + b)d$$

and if we apply it again to each of the two terms, the result for the binomial product is:

$$\boxed{(a + b)(c + d) = ac + bc + ad + bd} \qquad \text{Formula 3-2}$$

A particularly important special case of the binomial product is the square of a binomial, $(x + y)^2$. Because this is the same as $(x + y) \times (x + y)$, the rule for the binomial product, formula 3-2, can be applied to yield the following equation:

$$\boxed{(x + y)^2 = (x + y)(x + y) = x^2 + xy + xy + y^2 = x^2 + 2xy + y^2} \qquad \text{Formula 3-3}$$

Example 3-16. Find an expression without parentheses equal to $(p - q)^2$. In formula 3-3, x is replaced by p and y is replaced by $-q$. The result is $p^2 + 2p(-q) + (-q)^2 = p^2 - 2pq + q^2$.

Example 3-17. Give an expression without parentheses that is equal to $(2x - 3)^2$. By using formula 3-3 and changing x to $2x$ and y to -3 we obtain $(2x)^2 + 2(2x)(-3) + (-3)^2$, which is equal to $4x^2 - 12x + 9$.

FUNCTIONAL REPRESENTATION

Frequently there is a fixed relationship between two variables. If knowledge of the value of one variable permits the determination of the other, the relationship is called "functional." A *function* is that relationship between two variables in which the value of one variable can be found if the value of the other variable is known.

FUNCTIONAL RELATIONSHIP BETWEEN VARIABLES. Before discussing the formal relationship involved in functional notation we will consider a few examples.* The power P (in watts), associated with an electrical device is equal to the product of the current I (in amperes or amps) and the voltage V (in volts), or

$$P = IV$$

In fixed-voltage devices such as common electrical appliances, the power produced will depend on the current. For example, most general-purpose applications use 120 volts. A current of $\frac{1}{2}$ amp would result in 60 watts of power (suitable for a small lamp), 1 amp would produce a power of 120 watts, etc. It can be seen that the current determines the power. Or we can say that the power is a function of the current.

Another example is found in the transformation between the two most common temperature scales. Temperature is usually expressed in degrees of the Fahrenheit or Celsius (also called centigrade) scale. Let T_f stand for temperature measured on the Fahrenheit scale and T_c for temperature on the Celsius scale. If the first is known, the second can be found by the following relationship:

$$T_c = \frac{5(T_f - 32)}{9}$$

For example, when $T_f = 68°$, T_c is $20°$. We can say that the temperature in Celsius (T_c) is a function of the temperature in Fahrenheit. These two examples represent algebraic expressions of functional relationships between variables. Functional relationships can be expressed in other ways. One of these is by tabulation. An example is the common representation of the trigonometric functions discussed in Chapter 5. Another way of representing functions is by plotting a graph. Graphs and their interpretation are discussed in Chapter 6. By means of a graph we can obtain a specific value for one variable when the other is known or visualize the trend of one as the other changes.

---

*Many examples used in this text will be taken from radiological physics. Most of the formulas are for illustration only and the student is not expected to memorize them.

The notation for a functional relationship between the variables x and y is as follows:

$$y = f(x)$$

where y is a function of x; $f(x)$ is read "function of x" or "f of x." If we have another function of x, we can write it as $F(x)$ or $g(x)$, where F and g are symbols for different functions; which letters are used to indicate the function (F, g, etc.) is not important. What is important is that $F(x)$ or $g(x)$ in this context does *not* mean "F times x" or "g times x." For example, if $y = 1 - x^2$, we can express their relationship as $y = f(x)$ and $f(x) = 1 - x^2$.

Example 3-18. In Chapter 4 we will learn that the formula for determining the area of an equilateral triangle whose sides have a length s is $A = \dfrac{\sqrt{3}s^2}{4}$. If we write $A = f(s)$, what does $f(s)$ equal? The expression $f(s)$ must be equal to the expression involving s, or $f(s) = \dfrac{\sqrt{3}s^2}{4}$.

Sometimes we know that a functional relationship exists, but not exactly what it is. For example, we may know that a certain quantity q is a function of time (t). Instead of making the statement in words, we can write $q = T(t)$. But if we want to know the exact values, we must have certain details.

If a quantity, such as a dose (D), is a function of a variable, say time (t), we can write the function by using the variable's name: $D = D(t)$.

Example 3-19. Write the algebraic statement that the standard deviation σ of the number of counts (n) is a function of n. Use "σ" as the function symbol. Here the statement is written $\sigma = \sigma(n)$.

In the functional relationship $y = f(x)$, we call y the "dependent variable" and x the "independent variable." The implication is that y is determined when a value of x is assigned, whereas the value of x can be assigned arbitrarily.

It is conventional to write the dependent variable to the left and the expression involving the independent variable to the right.

Example 3-20. The formula for the temperature correction of ionization chamber readings is $C_T = \dfrac{(273 + T)}{295}$. Identify the independent variable. By the convention that the variable to the left is dependent and the one in the expression to the right is independent. T is called independent.

Functions of several variables. In many cases a quantity is related to several other quantities. For example, the exposure (X) from a fixed amount of radium or other radionuclide will increase as the time (t) increases, decrease as the distance (r) increases, and decrease as the thickness (x) of lead shielding increases. Without considering the precise relationship, we can say that the exposure is a function of t, r, and x. That is, for a fixed amount of a certain radioactive material there is a certain exposure X for a given t, r, and x. This can be written as $X = f(t,r,x)$. Note that all the variables are indicated in the functional notation. Here, t, r, and x are the independent variables and X is the single dependent variable.

> **Example 3-21.** In radiography, film density (D) can be considered as a function of the kilovoltage (kV), charge (mAs), filtration (f), focus-film distance (r), patient thickness (x), and screen-film speed (s). Write this with the dependent variable as the film density (D). This can be written as $D = H(kV,mAs,f,r,x,s)$, where H has been chosen as the symbol for the function.

> **Example 3-22.** The exposure X in milliroentgens (mR) from an un-shielded 10 mg of radium obeys the following formula:
>
> $$X(t,r) = 8.25 \frac{t}{r^2}$$
>
> where t is the time in hours and r is the distance in meters. What is $X(t = 20 \text{ min}, r = 10 \text{ cm})$? Convert 20 min to $\frac{1}{3}$ hour and 10 cm to 0.1 meter; thus $X(20 \text{ min}, 10 \text{ cm}) = X(\frac{1}{3}, 0.1) = 8.25 \, (\frac{1}{3}) \, (\frac{1}{0.1^2}) = 275$ mR.

> **Example 3-23.** A thimble chamber measurement of exposure yields a reading R. This reading must be corrected by a chamber factor C_c (supplied by a standardizing laboratory), a pressure correction $^{760}/_P$ (pressure P in mm Hg) and a temperature correction $\frac{(273 + T)}{295}$ (temperature T on the Celsius scale). The correct exposure (X) is:
>
> $$X(C_c,P,T,R) = C_c \, (^{760}/_P) \, \frac{(273 + T)}{295} (R)$$
>
> Find X if $C_c = 1.030$, $T = 24°$ C, $P = 755$ mm, and $R = 87$.
>
> $$X(1.030,755,24,87) = 1.030 \left(\frac{760}{755}\right) \left(\frac{273 + 24}{295}\right) 87 = 91$$

> **Example 3-24.** The number of counts (N) recorded by a detector is determined by the rate of particle emission $(n$, number per second$)$, the detection efficiency (E), and the time $(t$, in seconds$)$. N is the following function:
>
> $$N(n,E,t) = nEt$$

Find $N(3.7 \times 10^4, 0.031, 10)$. $N = 3.7 \times 10^4 \cdot 0.031 \cdot 10 = 1.1 \times 10^4$ counts.

EVALUATION OF FUNCTIONS. Sometimes we want to utilize the functional relationship to determine the dependent variable for a particular value (or group of values) of the independent variable. This was done for some of the examples in the previous two sections.

Consider an example. The effective half-life (T_E), of a radionuclide in the body is the time in which the activity of the radionuclide present in the body decreases to one half its initial value. The "effective half-life" is determined by the "physical half-life" $(T_P$, caused by nuclear decay), and by the "biological half-life" $(T_B$, caused by bodily elimination). The formula for the general case is $T_E = \dfrac{T_P T_B}{T_P + T_B}$. However, since the physical half-life remains constant for a given radionuclide (such as ^{99m}technetium [^{99m}Tc] with a physical life of 6 hours), the effective half-life becomes a function of the biological half-life only. For this example of ^{99m}Tc, the formula to obtain T_E is as follows:

$$T_E = f(T_B) = \frac{6T_B}{6 + T_B}$$

We can evaluate this function for various biological half-lives. If T_B is 3, T_E is evaluated as a function of 3: $T_E = f(3) = \dfrac{(6)3}{6 + 3} = \dfrac{18}{9} = 2$ hours. What is $f(6)$? Again the numerical value replaces T_B in the formula defining $f(T_B)$; the result is $f(6) = \dfrac{(6)6}{6 + 6} = \dfrac{36}{12} = 3$. In the same manner $f(4) = \dfrac{6(4)}{6 + 4} = \dfrac{24}{10} = 2.4$ hours.

The evaluation of a function or functional value results in a single number. The function represents a relationship for all legitimate values between the independent and the dependent variables; the evaluated function represents only one pair of values that satisfy the relationship.

Example 3-25. The uptake (U) of a thyroid gland expressed as a percent is given by the following formula:

$$U = f(C) = 100 \frac{(C - B)}{(C_A - B)}$$

where C is the number of counts in the patient (assume all counting times are one minute), B is the number of background counts, and C_A is the number of counts of the total administered radionuclide held in a suitable plastic phantom. If C_A is 7,000 and B is 1,000, evaluate $f(5,000)$. Now $f(C) = 100 \dfrac{(C - 1,000)}{(7,000 - 1,000)} = 100 \dfrac{(C - 1,000)}{6,000}$; thus

$f(5,000) = 100 \dfrac{4,000}{6,000} = 67\%$. In this example the functional value of the uptake, given that the number of counts is 5,000, results in a single number, 67%.

Example 3-26. In radiography, the width of the penumbra (W_p) is related to the width of the focal spot (W_s), the focus-film distance (FFD), and the object-film distance (d) by the following formula (developed in Chapter 4):

$$W_p = W_s \frac{d}{(FFD - d)}$$

For $FFD = 100$ cm (approximately the standard "table top" value) and $W_s = 1$ mm $= 0.1$ cm, the penumbra width is a function of the object-film distance: $W_p = f(d) = \dfrac{0.1d}{100 - d}$. Evaluate this for $f(5)$, $f(10)$, and $f(20)$.

$$f(5) = \frac{0.1\ (5)}{100 - 5} = \frac{0.5}{95} = 0.0053 \text{ cm}$$

$$f(10) = \frac{0.1\ (10)}{100 - 10} = \frac{1}{90} = 0.011 \text{ cm}$$

$$f(20) = \frac{0.1\ (20)}{100 - 20} = \frac{2}{80} = 0.025 \text{ cm}$$

A manipulation of functions that is very similar to evaluation is the substitution of one independent variable for another. For example, the circumference (C) of a circle (discussed in the next chapter) is a function of the diameter (d):

$$C = f(d) \cong 3.14d$$

If we wish to use the radius (r) of the circle rather than the diameter, we replace d by its equivalent, $2r$:

$$C = f(2r) \cong 3.14(2r) = 6.28r$$

Our result is now a function of the radius—but not the same function. Because 6.28 is not the same as 3.14, this is a different function and must receive a different designation, as follows:

$$C = F(r)$$

If we used $C = f(r)$, it would imply that $C = 3.14r$.

Example 3-27. In alternating-current electricity (AC), the power (P) in a resistance (R) is given by the formula $P = I^2R$, where I is the "root-mean-square" current. The root mean square (the square root of the mean of the squares) is an average of sorts, useful here because the current varies continuously with time. The root-mean-square current is related to the maximum current (I_m) by the formula $I = \dfrac{I_m}{\sqrt{2}}$. For a fixed resistance, say 100 ohms, the power is a function of the current:

$$P = g(I) = 100I^2$$

Express this in terms of the maximum current I_m. Replacing I by $\dfrac{I_m}{\sqrt{2}}$ we obtain the following:

$$P = g(I) = g\left(\frac{I_m}{\sqrt{2}}\right) = 100\left(\frac{I_m}{\sqrt{2}}\right)^2 = 100\,\frac{I_m^2}{2} = 50\,I_m^2$$

This can be represented as a new function:

$$P = G(I_m) = 50\,I_m^2$$

EQUATIONS

Several important tools of algebra have already been described. This section will deal with another one, the equation. At first it might appear that the equation is not very useful, but in reality it represents the single most powerful tool of algebra.

BASIC CONSIDERATIONS. Consider a function $f(x)$. The expression obtained by making it equal to 0 is

$$f(x) = 0 \qquad\qquad \textbf{Formula 3-5A}$$

and is called an *equation*. Besides this form, the equation may appear as follows:

$$f(x) = g(x) \qquad\qquad \textbf{Formula 3-5B}$$

Both formulas represent a condition on the variable x; the values of x must be such that $f(x)$ goes to zero in the first case or, in the second case, it makes the two values of the functions $f(x)$ and $g(x)$ equal. Any such value of x is called a *solution* of the equation under consideration. *Solving* the equation means finding all solutions. For example, in the equation $x + 2 = x^2$, there are two solutions, 2 and -1.

The equal sign used here has its usual meaning in mathematics and is read "is equal to." If one of the expressions in an equation is equal to a certain numerical value, the other expression cannot be equal to a different numerical value.*

If we have two equal quantities and perform the same operations on both of them, the two results are equal. This is true even if the quantities have a different appearance. For example, if we have equal quantities of water in two

---

*There are some other contexts in which the equal sign does not have the same meaning and in those contexts two expressions joined by an equal sign do not form an equation. For example, in the FORTRAN programming language for computers the statement $A = A + 1$ is perfectly legitimate, but it is certainly not an equation; the equal sign in FORTRAN is read "is replaced by."

containers, even though we may express the values in different units, one in milliliters and the other in kilograms, and equal amounts are withdrawn from each, then equal amounts remain in each container. This is the key to equations. We start with equality between two expressions and operate equally on each expression; the equality is preserved even though the form of the expressions may change considerably. We can perform several operations: we can add a number or an expression to both sides of an equation; subtract, multiply, or divide; take roots, squares, or the inverse; and even perform calculus operations.

Consider a sample equation: $6x - 3 = 3x + 3$. By adding 3 to both sides we obtain $6x - 3 + 3 = 3x + 3 + 3$ or $6x = 3x + 6$. This new equation is equivalent to the original equation in that the relationships and restrictions on the variable are unchanged, but the equation has a different appearance. Similarly, by subtracting $3x$ from both sides of the equation $6x = 3x + 6$, we obtain $6x - 3x = 3x + 6 - 3x$ or, simplified $3x = 6$. By dividing both sides of this result by 3, we obtain $3x \div 3 = 6 \div 3$, or $x = 2$. The number 2 is the only numerical value for x that will make the equation true. It is the value for x that gives the two expressions equal numerical value. The number 2 is called the "solution" of this equation. In subsequent sections of this chapter we will consider the problem of achieving solutions and special techniques in the manipulation of equations.

Let us manipulate the sample equation in a different way by substituting 2 for x and simplifying. The initial form of the equation $6x - 3 = 3x + 3$ becomes $9 = 9$. Adding 3 to both sides will yield $12 = 12$, which is the case when substituting 2 for x in $6x = 3x + 6$. Subtracting $3x$ from both sides is numerically equivalent to subtracting 6; this will yield $6 = 6$, which is indeed the value we obtain when $x = 2$ is applied to $3x = 6$. This numerical manipulation emphasizes how the original equality is maintained throughout the manipulations even though the values on both sides have changed.

Example 3-28. Subtract 2 from both sides of the equation $5x - 2 = 4x + 2$. The result is $5x - 2 - 2 = 4x + 2 - 2$ or $5x - 4 = 4x$.

Example 3-29. Square both sides of the equation $x + 1 = y - 1$. Using the results of the square of a binomial, formula 3-3, you will obtain $(x + 1)^2 = x^2 + 2x + 1$ and $(y - 1)^2 = y^2 - 2y + 1$; thus $x^2 + 2x + 1 = y^2 - 2y + 1$.

There are two things we must do if we are to use equations properly. First, we must begin with a true equality (we will discuss inequalities later in this chapter). Second, we must apply our operation correctly to both sides; some incorrect operations will be pointed out along the way.

Suppose we add 2 to both sides of the equation $x - 2 = \dfrac{x + 2}{2}$. The expression on the left becomes $x - 2 + 2$, or x. The right-hand expression is *not* $\dfrac{x+2+2}{2}$ *or* $\dfrac{x+4}{2}$ *but* $\dfrac{x+2}{2}+2=\dfrac{x+2}{2}+\dfrac{4}{2}=\dfrac{x+2+4}{2}=\dfrac{x+6}{2}$.

We must add 2 to the *expression,* not just to the *numerator.*

Suppose we divide $4y = 2x - 3$ by 2. The correct expressions are not $2y$ and $x - 3$, but $2y$ and $x - {}^3/_2$. A common mistake is to divide or multiply only a portion of the expression. Substituting a numerical value for x could help in detecting errors.

Similarly, roots, squaring, the operations of calculus, and other operations must be applied to the *entire* expression.

MANIPULATION OF EQUATIONS. We have seen that equations can be manipulated by applying the same mathematical operation to the two equal expressions. As a rule, we are interested in manipulations that yield a more useful form of the equation than the initial one, that is, a solution or a simpler equation. We shall analyze the effects of the more common manipulations before describing the methodical approach to obtaining a solution.

If one or both of the expressions in an equation contain a sum or a difference, it may be convenient to add or subtract an appropriate amount on both sides. For example, in the equation $2x = x - 3$ we might add 3 to both expressions to obtain $2x + 3 = x$. We might subtract x to obtain $x = -3$, we might subtract $2x$ to obtain $0 = -x - 3$, or we might subtract $x - 3$ from both sides to obtain $x + 3 = 0$. Careful analysis of the addition and subtraction processes yields an interesting shortcut. Consider the following equation:

$$x + y = z$$

Subtract y from both sides. The equation becomes

$$x = z - y$$

Comparing these two forms we see that y, the quantity subtracted, appears to move from one side of the equal sign to the other with a change of sign.

> **Example 3-30.** Remove $2x$ from the left-hand side of the equation $2x - 3 = 4x - 7$ by appropriate means. We can move it by subtracting $2x$ from both sides, yielding $-3 = 4x - 2x - 7$, or $-3 = 2x - 7$.

A useful shortcut is moving an expression to the other side of the equal sign. But remember that when you do this, you must change the sign of the expression.

Multiplication is particularly useful in the case of equations involving fractions. For example, the equation

$$\frac{x+1}{x} = \frac{3x-1}{2x}$$

can be simplified to $2(x + 1) = 3x - 1$ by multiplying both sides by $2x$.

> **Example 3-31.** Multiply the equation $\dfrac{x+1}{x} = \dfrac{2x-1}{2}$ by $2x$. The

equation becomes $\dfrac{2x(x + 1)}{x} = \dfrac{2x(2x - 1)}{2}$, or canceling common factors, $2(x + 1) = x(2x - 1)$, or $2x + 2 = 2x^2 - x$ by clearing the parentheses.

By what factor should a particular equation be multiplied to eliminate the denominators? Let us assume that an equation can be written as $N/D = n/d$. If we multiply this equation by the denominator on the left, D, we will eliminate the left denominator. The equation will be $N = nD/d$. Now multiplying by the denominator on the right, d, we eliminate that denominator as well; the equation is now $Nd = nD$. The two multiplications can be reduced to one by multiplying by both denominators at once, in this case dD.

Example 3-32. What should the equation $\dfrac{x^2 - y^2}{1 + x} = \dfrac{2xy}{1 - y}$ be multiplied by to eliminate the denominators? Because the denominators are $1 + x$ and $1 - y$, multiplying by $(1 + x)(1 - y)$ will eliminate both denominators.

The shortcut for multiplication is illustrated by the method we used to manipulate the equation $N/D = n/d$; with the denominators eliminated, this becomes $Nd = nD$. The denominators appear to cross the equal sign and go into the numerator on the opposite side. This shortcut is called "cross multiplication."

Division is useful if there is a common factor on both sides. For example, in the equation $3x(2x + 1) = 3x(x - 2)$ we can divide both sides by $3x$ to obtain $2x + 1 = x - 2$, obviously a simpler form than before.

Example 3-33. Factor the equation $6x^2 + 4x = 9x^2 + 3x$ and eliminate any factors common to both sides by division. Common factors in the left-hand expression are 2 and x. The common factors to the right are 3 and x. The equation can be written $2x(3x + 2) = 3x(3x + 1)$. The factor common to both sides is x; division by x yields the equation $2(3x + 2) = 3(3x + 1)$.

Keep in mind that when dividing an equation to eliminate a common factor that contains the variables you will lose a solution. For instance, in the equation $3x(2 + 1) = 3x(x - 2)$ there are two possible solutions, $x = 0$ or $x = -3$. But if you eliminate the common factor $3x$, the remaining equation, $2x + 1 = x - 2$, yields only one solution, $x = -3$.

There are other useful manipulations. Equations involving radicals (terms under a root sign), such as $\sqrt{a}$, can sometimes be simplified by appropriate squaring, cubing, and so forth. Equations of high power can occasionally be simplified by taking a root. Here remember that square roots come in pairs—a positive one and a negative one.

Solution of simple equations. An equation can be viewed as a scale that will balance only if both sides carry equal weights—the relationship of equality between expressions. To ensure this equality, there must obviously be restrictions on the values that variables can take. Whenever we express the condition implied by the equal sign on a certain variable, say x, as x = terms not involving x, then we have a "solution of the equation" for x. For example, $x = 4y + 3$. If x is the only variable in the equation, this solution is a number, as in $x = 4$. As shown in the previous section, there may be more than one solution to an equation. We will now look at ways to solve an equation.

"Solutions" may be expressed in terms of variables when there are several variables in the equation. The solution still has the form of one variable being equal to an expression that generally involves the other variables. Earlier, the equation for the temperature in Celsius (T_c) in terms of temperature in Fahrenheit (T_f) was given as follows:

$$T_c = \frac{5(T_f - 32)}{9}$$

This form is a solution of the equation for T_c. Using the operations described previously in the discussion of manipulation of equations, it can be transformed to the form $T_f = \dfrac{9T_c}{5} + 32$. This can be called the solution of the equation for T_f.

> **Example 3-34.** The formula for the temperature correction of ionization chambers (C_t) in terms of the temperature in Celsius (T) is $C_t = \dfrac{273 + T}{295}$. Solve this equation for T. Multiply both sides by 295 and subtract 273 from both sides; this leaves $295C_t - 273 = T$, or reversed, $T = 295C_t - 273$.

We can test a solution by substituting it in the original equation. This is a good general practice.

> **Example 3-35.** Verify by substitution that -3 is a solution of the equation $3x(2x + 1) = 3x(x - 2)$. Substituting -3 for x yields $3(-3)[2(-3) + 1] = 3(-3)(-3 - 2)$, or $-9(-6 + 1) = -9(-5)$, or $-9(-5) = +45$, or $45 = 45$. This shows that -3 is a solution.

If we are told that the solution to $x + 1 = 3x - 1$ may be -1, 0, or $+1$, we might hazard a guess (and then verify) that the correct answer is $+1$. Good guessing, of course, requires either good luck or experience. However, to find a solution in a methodical way is probably most efficient. There are many methods for solving equations; the following sequence is one possible approach.

First, *eliminate the denominators* by appropriate multiplication.

Second, *eliminate any roots* by taking the appropriate power. For example, in the equation $\sqrt{x} = 1 + y$ the square root can be eliminated by squaring both sides to obtain $x = (1 + y)^2$.

Third, *eliminate all parentheses* by appropriate operations.

Fourth, *collect like terms*. If there is a single variable, it is conventional to place it to the left of the equal sign and the constants to the right. If there are several variables, one dependent variable is placed to the left of the equal sign and all the other variables and constants are placed to the right.

Fifth, if possible, *carry out the necessary operation* (such as division) to obtain the result in the form of a solution.

Finally, *check the solution* by substituting it into the equation.

Example 3-36. Solve the equation $5 = \dfrac{(1 + y)}{(1 - y)}$ by using the sequence of operations just discussed. First, eliminate the denominator by multiplying both sides by $1 - y$. The result is $5(1 - y) = (1 + y)$. The second step is not applicable, since there are no roots. Carry out the third step by using the distributive law. The result is $5 - 5y = 1 + y$. In the fourth step collect the y terms to the left by subtracting y and 5 from both sides. This yields $-5y - y = 1 - 5$, which is simplified to $-6y = -4$. Perform the fifth step, dividing the equation by -6. The result is $y = \frac{2}{3}$. Finally, substitute this solution in the original equation: $5 = (1 + \frac{2}{3}) \div (1 - \frac{2}{3})$; or $5 = (\frac{5}{3}) \div (\frac{1}{3})$; or $5 = 5$. This shows that our solution is correct.

Example 3-37. Solve the equation $y = \dfrac{1}{\sqrt{1 - x^2}}$ for x by using the same procedure.

Step 1 $\quad y\sqrt{1 - x^2} = 1$

Step 2 $\quad y^2(1 - x^2) = 1$

Step 3 $\quad y^2 - y^2 x^2 = 1$

Step 4 $\quad -y^2 x^2 = 1 - y^2$

Step 5 $\quad x = \pm\sqrt{\dfrac{(y^2 - 1)}{y^2}}$

Step 6 $\quad y = \dfrac{1}{\sqrt{1 - \dfrac{(y^2 - 1)}{y^2}}} = \dfrac{1}{\sqrt{\dfrac{(y^2 - y^2 + 1)}{y^2}}} = \dfrac{1}{\sqrt{\dfrac{1}{y^2}}} = \dfrac{1}{(\frac{1}{y})} = y$

Notice the two solutions of x: $+\sqrt{\dfrac{(y^2 - 1)}{y^2}}$ and $-\sqrt{\dfrac{(y^2 - 1)}{y^2}}$.

Frequently there is a common factor on both sides of the equal sign. Although factoring was not included in the steps enumerated, it should be used whenever possible.

Equations are called linear, quadratic, cubic, etc., depending on the *highest* power of the variable present after step 4. If x is the highest variable, the equation is linear; if x^2, it is quadratic; if x^3, cubic; and so forth. In general, linear equations have one solution, quadratic equations have two, and cubic equations have three. Linear equations can always be solved readily with the methods described. Quadratic equations, if they contain no linear term, are also easily solved, as in the last example. In general, quadratic equations can be written in the form $Ax^2 + Bx + C = 0$, where A, B, and C are constants. A general solution to this is the "quadratic" formula:

$$x = \frac{-B \pm \sqrt{B^2 - 4AC}}{2A}$$

Formula 3-6

The two solutions correspond to the two signs in front of the radical.

Example 3-38. Solve the equation $x + 3 = (x + 1)(x - 2)$. First eliminate the parentheses; the result is $x + 3 = x^2 + x - 2x - 2$. By collecting like terms to the left of the equation it becomes $-x^2 + 2x + 5 = 0$. The quadratic formula is now applied as $x = \dfrac{-2 \pm \sqrt{4 + 20}}{-2}$ $= \dfrac{+2 \pm \sqrt{24}}{2} = 1 \pm \sqrt{6}$. The two solutions are $1 - \sqrt{6} \cong -1.45$ and $1 + \sqrt{6} \cong 3.45$. As approximate decimals, they can be checked on a calculator.

A formula for cubic equations can be found in standard mathematical handbooks. There is no general formula for higher order equations.

EQUATIONS IN WORDS. Many mathematical problems can be formulated as equations. The wording can usually be translated into algebraic expressions and their relationship, and this, in turn, can often be represented as an equality. Here is a typical problem suitable for analysis as an equation: "Two vials contain technetium. Vial A contains 50% more than vial B. Together they contain 22 mCi. How much is in each vial?" This can be set up algebraically as follows: First, define the amount in vial B as q. The amount in A is then $1.5q$. Now we want the total amount (the word "together" implies addition). In terms of "q" the total amount $(A + B)$ is $1.5q + q$. The other expression is the 22 mCi. Thus the equation is $1.5q + q = 22$.

Example 3-39. A certain radium stock consists of three source strengths. Type 2 is 50% stronger than type 1 and type 3 is $2\frac{1}{2}$ times as strong as type 1. There are four type 1, eight type 2, and two type 3 sources in the stock. The total strength is 42 mg. Write an equation for the strength of type 1 sources. Let the strength for type 1 be s. Type 2 is then $1.5s$ and type 3 strength is $2.5s$. The total amount is $4s + 8(1.5s) + 2(2.5s) = 42$.

Example 3-40. On a certain day, radiographer A took twelve more films than radiographer B. Radiographer B's share of the combined films was 45%. Write this as an equation. Let N equal the number that B took. Then N is equal to 45% (0.45) of the total; the total is the number A took ($N + 12$) plus those B took (N) or $N + 12 + N$. Thus the equation is $N = 0.45(N + 12 + N)$.

Once an equation is set up, we can solve it by the methods already discussed.

INEQUALITIES

Inequalities are similar to equations in that they represent a relationship between expressions. However, this relationship is one of "greater than" or "less than" and is much less restrictive with respect to the variables involved than an equation.

Inequalities are especially useful where we wish to indicate the range of values that satisfy a certain condition, such as the validity of a certain formula or another inequality. For example, we can say that positive numbers are those numbers that are greater than zero.

INEQUALITY SYMBOLS. The relationships "greater than" and "less than" are expressed by the symbols ">" and "<," respectively. For example, $A > B$ is read "A is greater than B" and $x - 1 < x^2$ is read "x minus 1 is less than x^2."

There are other symbols used in inequalities. The two just mentioned can be combined with the "equal" sign thus: "≤" and "≥"; they are read as "less than or equal to" and as "greater than or equal to." The symbol $\neq$ means "not equal to." See the boxed material on this page for additional symbols.

Inequalities may be used to express a condition of certain variables; for example, if x is always positive, we write $x > 0$; if P never exceeds 100, but might equal 100, we write $P \leq 100$. A range of values limited on both sides can be indicated by two inequalities; for example, if I is less than or equal to I_0, but always greater than 0, we can write $0 < I$ and $I \leq I_0$. Note that $0 < I$

SYMBOLS USED IN INEQUALITIES

Symbol	Word meaning
$>$	Greater than
$<$	Less than
$\geq$	Greater than or equal to
$\leq$	Less than or equal to
$\gtrsim$	Greater than or approximately equal to
$\lesssim$	Less than or approximately equal to
$>>$	Much greater than
$<<$	Much less than
$\neq$	Not equal to

is the same as $I > 0$. A pair of inequalities dealing with the same variable or expression is often written as one double relationship; for example $0 < I$ and $I \leq I_0$ can be written $0 < I \leq I_0$.

If a numerical value fits the specified conditions, it is said to "satisfy" the inequality. For example, if $0 < I < I_0$, then I values of $(^1/_{10})I_0$, $(^2/_3)I_0$, or $\sqrt{^2/_3}$ I_0 would all satisfy the inequality; the values $I = -\dfrac{I_0}{2}$, $3I_0$, or $\sqrt{2}I_0$ would not satisfy it. Because there are many values that may satisfy an inequality, guessing is not as helpful here as with equations.

OPERATIONS WITH INEQUALITIES. If an inequality contains some fairly complicated expressions, it may be necessary to simplify them in order to find the solutions that satisfy it. For example, $x^2 - 1 < 1$ can be simplified to $-\sqrt{2} < x < \sqrt{2}$, which readily indicates that the values of x must be greater than $-\sqrt{2}$ and less than $+\sqrt{2}$ to satisfy the inequality.

The legitimate manipulations of inequalities are similar to those of equations but require a few additional rules. If $x = y$, it is also true that $y = x$. However, to reverse the order of an inequality we must also reverse the inequality symbol (except in the case of the more general "not equal," which will not be considered here). For example: if $w > z$, then $z < w$, *not $z > w$.*

If equal quantities are added to or subtracted from both sides, the inequality is preserved. For example, if $C > D$, then $C + x > D + x$. This will allow us to collect terms in a manner similar to that used with equations.

> **Example 3-41.** In the inequality $x + 4 < 2x - 3$, group all terms involving x to the left and all purely numerical terms to the right. First, we subtract 4 from both sides to obtain $x < 2x - 7$. Then we subtract $2x$ from both sides; the result is $-x < -7$.

Multiplication or division by a *negative* number will reverse the inequality. Whereas 5 is less than 10, -5 is greater than -10. Multiplication or division by a *positive* number will not reverse the inequality. Thus if we multiply $x < -1$ by 2, we obtain $2x < -2$; but if we multiply it by -1, we obtain $-x > +1$.

> **Example 3-42.** Multiply $-x < -7$ by -1. The answer is $(-1)(-x) > (-1)(-7)$, or $x > 7$.

Powers and roots must be manipulated very carefully, since the inequality signs may be reversed by certain operations. The inequality $x^2 < 9$ is not equivalent to $x < 3$; for example if the value of x is -4, the second inequality would be satisfied, but the first would not.

CHAPTER REVIEW

1. What does an unknown represent?
2. Why is it sometimes convenient to use variables?
3. What is an expression?
4. Why are parentheses used in expressions?
5. What is factoring?
6. What is a binomial?
7. What is a binomial product?
8. What is a dependent variable? What is its relationship to a function?
9. How is a function evaluated?
10. How are expressions and equations related?
11. What is the basic rule for manipulating equations?
12. What is the solution of an equation?
13. Are solutions always numerical?
14. What is the order of manipulations in solving an equation?
15. What is the quadratic formula and when is it used?
16. What are inequalities used for?
17. Are there solutions to inequalities?

PROBLEMS
Problems paralleling chapter examples

1. **(3-1)** A patient, who has already received a dose of d_0 rads, will today receive an additional 200 rads. What will the total dose be after today's treatment?
2. **(3-2)** Express $(x + 1) - (2x - 1)$ without parentheses.
3. **(3-3)** Evaluate the expression $x - 2y$ when $x = 3$ and $y = 1$.
4. **(3-6)** Collect the terms in the expression $(5x + 1) - (x + y) + (2y - x)$.
5. **(3-8)** Group by power the terms of the expression $x + 5 - xy + x^2 - y$.
6. **(3-10)** Find the common factor in $x^4y + xy^4$ and factor it out.
7. **(3-13)** Subtract x/y from $\dfrac{(x + 1)}{(y + 1)}$.
8. **(3-16)** Express $(p + 2q)^2$ without parentheses.
9. **(3-19)** Write the algebraic statement that the chamber temperature correction

(C_t) is a function of the temperature (T).

10. **(3-20)** The area of a square with sides of length l is $A = l^2$. Which variable, A or l, would we call dependent?
11. **(3-21)** The activity (A) remaining in a vial of radiopharmaceuticals depends on the initial activity (A_o), the elapsed time (t), the decay constant (λ), and the fraction of solution removed (f). Write the dependent variable as a function (q) of the independent variables.
12. **(3-22)** The exposure $(X$, in milliroentgens) at a distance $(r$, in meters) from 20 mg of radium encapsulated by 0.5 mm of platinum is $X(r, t) = \dfrac{16.5t}{r^2}$, where t is the time in hours. Find $X(r = 10$ cm, $t = 20$ min) and $X(3$ meters, 2 days).
13. **(3-23)** The correct exposure is $X(C_c,$
$$P, \ T, \ R) = \left[C_c \ \frac{(760/P)(273 + T)}{295} \right] R.$$
Here, C_c is the chamber correction factor, P the pressure in millimeters of mercury, T the temperature in degrees Celsius, and R the chamber reading. Find $X(0.98, 757, 26, 59)$ and $X(0.94, 762, 18, 61)$.
14. **(3-24)** If $N(n, E, t) = nEt$, find $N(6 \times 10^{12}, 0.0047, 5)$.
15. **(3-25)** If $U = f(C) = \dfrac{100(C - B)}{C_A - B}$ and $C_A = 11{,}000$ and $B = 1{,}000$, evaluate $f(6{,}000)$ and $f(2{,}000)$.
16. **(3-26)** The formula for the width of the penumbra (W_p), in terms of the focal-spot width (W), the focus-film distance (FFD), and the object-film distance (d), is $W_p = f(d)$ where $f(d) = \dfrac{d \cdot W}{FFD - d}$, for an FFD of 180 cm and a focal-spot width of 0.2 cm, find $f(5)$ and $f(10)$.
17. **(3-27)** The temperature correction for an ionization chamber reading is $C_t = f(T_c) = \dfrac{T_c + 273}{295}$. The relation-

ship between the temperature on the Celsius scale (T_c) and the temperature on the Fahrenheit scale (T_f) is $T_c = \frac{5}{9}(T_f - 32)$. Find $F(T_f)$ where $C_t = F(T_f)$.

18. **(3-28)** Remove the purely numerical term from the left-hand side of the equation $2x - 3 = 4x - 7$ by an appropriate operation.

19. **(3-30)** Subtract $4x$ from both sides of the equation $5x - 2 = 4x + 2$.

20. **(3-31)** Multiply the equation $\frac{x+1}{x} = \frac{x+1}{x-1}$ by $x(x-1)$ and cancel any common factors remaining.

21. **(3-32)** By what should the equation $\frac{A+3}{A+B} = \frac{A-B}{B}$ be multiplied to eliminate the denominator?

22. **(3-33)** Factor each expression in the equation $4ax^2 + 12a^3x = 6a^2x^2 + 18ax$ as much as possible without creating any denominators. Cancel any factors common to both sides of the equation.

23. **(3-34)** Solve the equation $N = nEt$ for E.

24. **(3-35)** Verify that $+4$ is not a solution to the equation $3x(2x + 1) = 3x(x - 2)$.

25. **(3-36)** Solve the equation $4 = \frac{s}{s-1}$.

26. **(3-37)** Solve the equation $\frac{1}{\sqrt{1-v^2/c^2}} = 1.5$ for v. Assume v and c are positive.

27. **(3-38)** Solve the equation $x + 2 = (x + 4)(x + 1)$.

28. **(3-39)** A technician withdrew some fluid from vial A and some from vial B in the ratio 3:5; the total withdrawn was 1 ml. Write an equation using the volume (v) withdrawn from vial A as the variable.

29. **(3-40)** Two carts are loaded with standard lead bricks. One cart has 5 more bricks than the other; the cart with more bricks has 60% of the total. Write an equation for the total number of bricks in terms of "n," the number on the cart with more bricks.

30. **(3-41)** Collect the terms in the following inequality so that terms involving A are to the left and those involving B are to the right: $2A + 3B > A + 2$.

31. **(3-42)** Multiply $y + 2 < z - 1$ by -1.

Problems related to this chapter

32. For an object at a distance (d) from a film with a focal film distance of 100 cm, the magnification (M) is $M(d) = 1 + \frac{d}{100 - d}$. Evaluate this function for $d = 10, 20,$ and 30 cm.

33. For a pure radioactive material, the activity $(A,$ the number of disintegrations per second) obeys the approximate formula (short times) $A(t) = A_0(1 - \lambda t)$, where A_0 is the initial activity, λ the decay constant, and t the time. For the situation in which $A_0 = 50$ mCi and $\lambda = 0.115$ hr^{-1} (corresponding to the six-hour half-life of ^{99m}Tc), find $A(0), A(\frac{1}{2}), A(1),$ and $A(2)$.

34. Evaluate the expression $(N - 3)^2$ when $N = 5$.

35. Express the following without parentheses:
   a. $3(a-b)$
   b. $(a + b) - (2a + b)$
   c. $(a + b)^2$
   d. $(6a - 4b) \div 2$
   e. $(2 - 3x)(4x + 1)$

36. Evaluate the function indicated for the specified value of the variables. Example: $f(x) = x^2 - 1$ for $x = 3$ gives $f(3) = 8$.
   a. $f(x) = 1 + 3x$ for $x = 4$
   b. $g(x) = \frac{1-x}{1-x}$ for $x = 2$
   c. $F(x) = 1 - x$ for $x = u + 1$
   d. $f(x) = x^3 - x$: find $f(0)$

37. Collect terms in the equation $2x - 3 = 6x + 1$ in the conventional manner.

38. Solve the following equations for y:
   a. $y + 2 = -3$
   b. $6y + 7 = y + 21$
   c. $4y^2 = 16$
   d. $\frac{y+1}{y} = 2$
   e. $\frac{1}{y} = 10$
   f. $2x - 6y = 12$

39. Solve the following equations for x in terms of y. Example: $y = x - 3$; solution: $x = y + 3$.
   a. $y = 2x$
   b. $y = 6x - 2$
   c. $y = \frac{2}{x}$
   d. $y = \frac{2}{x + 3}$
   e. $y = \frac{x+1}{x-1}$

40. Solve the following equations for the unknown indicated in each case.

    a. $x + 3 = \dfrac{x}{2} - 1$

    b. $3(y - 3) = 2(y + 1)$

    c. $\dfrac{1}{x} - 1 = \dfrac{2}{x + 3}$ (two solutions)

    d. $t^2 - t = 2t$ (two solutions)

    e. $\dfrac{3z + 1}{4z - 1} = 5$

41. What is the largest value x can have if $3 > (1 - x) \geq 1$.

42. What is the smallest value y can have if $0 < 2y < 5$.

Formulate the next 6 questions as algebraic statements: the solution is optional.

43. At a certain time a technician counts the number of patients (x) waiting for processing. During the next hour, four more patients arrive and seven are processed and leave. The technician sees that there are now half as many patients waiting. On the left of the equation below write the number of patients (using x) that are calculated to be present at the end of the hour, accounting for the number that came and went. On the right use the calculation based on the second count.

    _____ = _____

44. The area of a rectangle is its length (l) multiplied by its width (w). A certain rectangle has a length three times longer than its width. The area is 12 cm². Write the formula for the area in terms of w to the left of the equal sign and the numerical value to the right.

    _____ = _____

45. Technician A and technician B produce the same total of good films each day (call this number "n"). For every 10 acceptable films, technician A produces an average of 1 waste film (one "retake"); technician B produces 2 waste films for every 10 usable films on the average. At the end of the average day the two technicians have produced a total of 36 waste films. Equate the calculated number of waste films (using n) on the left with the count on the right.

    _____ = _____

46. A detector is first used to count the background count rate. In one minute it counts a certain number (N). The sample is put in place and the total count is found to be $7\frac{1}{2}$ times the background. The net count is equal to the total count less the background. The net count is found to be 11,256 counts. Equate this net count (in terms of N) with this number.

    _____ = _____

47. In processing some paper work, the clerk notes that about $\frac{1}{3}$ of the forms have been filled. After filling out ten more forms, he sees about $\frac{1}{2}$ of the forms have been completed. Call the total number of forms x and equate the two evaluations of the number of forms completed.

    _____ = _____

Objective questions

Find the correct answer.

48. If $x = 2 - u$ and $y = 2x - 1$, then we can also write y as:

    a. $3 - 2u$

    b. $2u + 5$

    c. $3 - u$

    d. $2u + 3$

    e. $u - 1$

49. If $x = 1 + 16t^2$ (x and t positive), then t is equal to:

    a. $\dfrac{x^2 - 1}{16}$

    b. $\sqrt{\dfrac{x}{16} - 1}$

    c. $\dfrac{2x - 1}{16}$

    d. $\sqrt{\dfrac{x - 1}{16}}$

    e. $\dfrac{x - 1}{16} - 2$

50. If $y = 2x^2$, which of the following is not true:

    a. $y^2 = 4x^4$

    b. $^{y}/_{2} = x^2$

    c. $y + 4 = 2(x^2 + 2)$

    d. $y^2 = 2x$

51. If $y = x^3$ and $x = 2$, then y is:

    a. 1

    b. 6

    c. 8

    d. 9

52. If $x + 7 = 3x - 1$, then x equals:

    a. 1   d. 4

    b. 2   e. 8

    c. 3

53. If $v = \sqrt{\dfrac{2(E - V)}{m}}$, then E is equal to:

    a. $\sqrt{\dfrac{2(v - V)}{m}}$

    b. $\dfrac{1}{2} mv^2 + V$

    c. $\dfrac{1}{2m(v^2 + V)}$

    d. $\dfrac{2(\sqrt{v} - V)}{m}$

    e. $(V - v)2m$

54. The relationship $2x + 4 > x - 4$ is equivalent to:

    a. $x > -8$

    b. $x > -4$

    c. $x > 0$

    d. $x > +4$

    e. $x > +8$

55. The equation $(x + 1)(x + 2) = x + 3$ is known as:

    a. a linear equation

    b. a quadratic equation

    c. a cubic equation

    d. all of the above

    e. none of the above

56. The equation $x^2 - 5x + 6 = 0$ has:

    a. no solutions

    b. the single solution $x = 2$

    c. the pair of solutions $x = 2$ and $x = 3$

    d. an unlimited number of solutions

57. An operation that we cannot perform on an equation is:

    a. adding 6 to both sides

    b. subtracting 4 from both sides

    c. multiplying by -1

    d. dividing by zero

    e. squaring both sides

58. In the "solved equation" $y = 2x + 1$ the variables x and y are called _____ and _____, respectively:

    a. dependent, dependent

    b. dependent, independent

    c. independent, independent

    d. independent

CHAPTER 4

Geometry

Geometry is the science that deals with the relationship between points, lines, and angles. Here we will be concerned primarily with straight lines in a two-dimensional space; this means that most of our figures can be drawn with a straight edge on a sheet of paper. Occasionally, we will consider aspects of circles, arcs of circles, and three-dimensional forms.

ANGLES

When two lines intersect (join or cross), they form an *angle*. If one of the lines is horizontal and to the right of the vertex, the angle it forms with another line is measured in a counterclockwise direction; this angle is in standard position. Such an angle is shown in Fig. 4-1.

Several schemes for measuring angles exist. The oldest and most common method is to divide a complete revolution into 360 degrees. Then a *right angle,* which is one fourth of a complete revolution, is 90 degrees. Two adjacent right angles, or a "straight angle," is 180 degrees. These angles are shown in Fig. 4-2. Often a right angle is indicated in short form as shown in Fig. 4-3.

DEGREES AND RADIANS. Angles are almost always measured in *degrees*.* The simplest device for angle measurements is the *protractor;* its form and use is shown in Fig. 4-4. For measurements of fractions of a degree, decimals can be used. The degree can also be divided into sixty minutes and the minute into sixty seconds.

> **Example 4-1.** Express 17°35′ as a decimal. If $^{35}/_{60} = 0.58$, 35 minutes equals 0.58° and 17°35′ = 17.58 degrees.

> **Example 4-2.** Express 0.33 degree in minutes. Since there are 60 minutes in a degree, 0.33 degree is $0.33 \times 60 = 20'$. (Here the 19.8 minutes have been rounded to 20 minutes.)

Angles of interest to radiologists rarely require precision beyond degrees. The examples given would most likely be used in connection with trigonometric tables discussed in the next chapter.

A much less common unit for angle measurements is the *radian*. This can

---

*Officially, the International System of Units (SI) measures angles using the "grad"; 100 grads equals a right angle. This unit has never received wide acceptance and is almost never used.

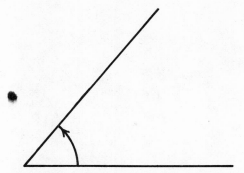

Fig. 4-1. An angle in standard position. Angles are measured from a horizontal line to the right of the vertex. The positive direction for angles is counterclockwise (to the left).

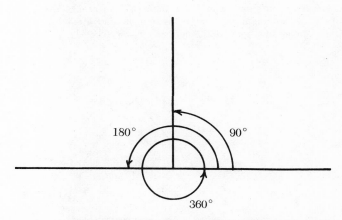

Fig. 4-2. Special angles. A right angle is 90 degrees, a straight angle (or half revolution) is 180 degrees, and a full revolution is 360 degrees.

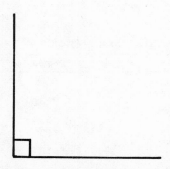

Fig. 4-3. A right angle is often indicated by a small square drawn in the angle.

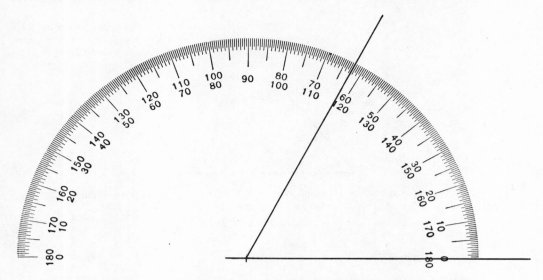

Fig. 4-4. Angle measurement with a protractor. The protractor base is placed along one of the lines with the center line at the vertex. The angle is read where the other line crosses the curved scale. The angle shown here is 62.5 degrees.

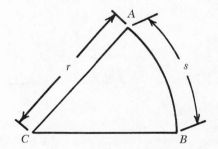

Fig. 4-5. Radian measure. The figure *ABC* represents an arc *AB* of length *s,* and an angle with vertex at *C,* the center of a circle whose radius *r* is the distance *CB = CA.* Regardless of the radius chosen, the ratio *s/r* is constant for any given angle. This ratio is the "radians" of the angle.

Table 2
Measurements of some common angles

Name	Degrees	Radians
Full revolution	360°	2π
Half revolution Straight angle	180°	
—	135°	$3\pi/4$
Right angle	90°	$\pi/2$
	60°	$\pi/3$
—	45°	$\pi/4$
—	30°	$\pi/6$

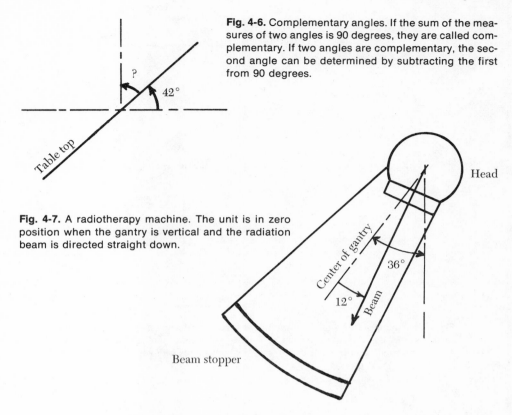

Fig. 4-6. Complementary angles. If the sum of the measures of two angles is 90 degrees, they are called complementary. If two angles are complementary, the second angle can be determined by subtracting the first from 90 degrees.

Fig. 4-7. A radiotherapy machine. The unit is in zero position when the gantry is vertical and the radiation beam is directed straight down.

be defined in geometric terms as the ratio between arc and radius, as is shown in Fig. 4-5. We can also say that a complete revolution is the angle 2π radians; π (pi) is the ratio of the circumference of a circle to the diameter (approximately $\pi \cong 3.14$). In most applications, radians are expressed as multiples of π. Some common angles are indicated in Table 2 on p. 62. For common angles such as the right angle, the radian and the degree values are often used interchangeably.

If the sum of the measures of two angles is 90 degrees, they are called *complementary*. If two angles are complementary, the second angle can be determined by subtracting the first from 90 degrees.

> **Example 4-3.** A patient table is tilted 42 degrees with respect to the horizontal (see Fig. 4-6). What is the angle with respect to the vertical? The horizontal and vertical lines form a right angle, or 90 degrees; hence the angle between the table and the vertical is $90° - 42° = 48°$.

> **Example 4-4.** If the gantry of a radiotherapy machine is tilted 36 degrees and the therapy head is angled 12 degrees with respect to the gantry, as shown in Fig. 4-7, what is the angle between the beam direction and the vertical? The angle is $36° - 12° = 24°$.

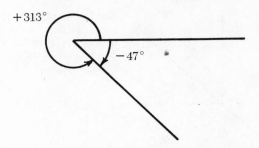

Fig. 4-8. A negative angle. This angle (measured clockwise) is −47 degrees.

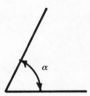

Fig. 4-9. The magnitude of an angle. If we are only interested in the size of an angle and not in whether it is measured clockwise or counterclockwise, we can indicate this with the double arrow as shown, by omitting the arrows, or sometimes by even omitting the arc.

Angles of unspecified or unknown size are usually indicated by letters. Small Greek letters, particularly α (alpha), β (beta), γ (gamma), θ (theta), and ϕ (phi) are the most common used. Occasionally, small or capital Roman letters are used.

OTHER TERMS. An angle measured clockwise is called *negative* (Fig. 4-8). It can be expressed as a *positive* angle by adding 360 degrees to it. For example −90 degrees describes the same angle as +270 degrees. Note that moving a particular device 90 degrees clockwise results in the same position as moving it 270 degrees counterclockwise; of course, the amount of motion is not the same. Often we are not interested in the direction or sense in which an angle is measured but only in its size or magnitude. In this case the angle is always expressed as positive, but the arc indicating the angle is given arrows pointing in both directions, as shown in Fig. 4-9.

Angles that are smaller than 90 degrees are called *acute;* those greater than 90 degrees are called *obtuse*.

When two straight lines intersect, they form four angles (α, β, θ, and ϕ in Fig. 4-10). From the fact that the lines are straight it can be seen that:

$$\alpha + \beta = 180° = \alpha + \theta = \theta + \phi = \phi + \beta \qquad \text{Formula 4-1}$$

These relations imply that

$$\alpha = \phi; \beta = \theta \qquad \text{Formula 4-2}$$

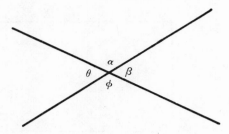

Fig. 4-10. Two intersecting straight lines. Since $\alpha + \beta = 180°$, $\theta + \phi = 180°$, $\theta + \alpha = 180°$ and $\phi + \beta = 180°$, the opposite angles must be equal, that is, $\alpha = \phi$ and $\beta = \theta$.

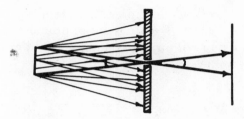

Fig. 4-11. The pinhole camera for x rays. A small hole in lead sheet makes a pinhole camera for x rays. For the rays drawn heavily, the angle to the left of the pinhole must equal the angle to the right.

This means: *When two straight lines intersect, the opposite angles are of equal magnitude.* To describe this situation, the size of the acute angle is usually given. An example of its use is given in Fig. 4-11. When the sum of two angles equals 180 degrees, the two angles are called *supplementary.* For example, in Fig. 4-10, α and β, α and θ, θ and ϕ, and ϕ and β are all pairs of supplementary angles.

TWO-DIMENSIONAL GEOMETRIC FIGURES

Geometric figures can be conceived of as combinations of lines and angles. Most of the figures that we will use are formed by straight lines, and most are "closed." A closed figure is one that ends at the starting point, as in a square.

In analyzing a geometric figure, we may generate new ones, which are easier to interpret, by adding lines. These lines are often *normal* (at right angles to a line), *parallel* (straight lines that will not intersect no matter how far they are extended), or *bisecting* (lines that divide angles or other line segments in half).

THE RECTANGLE. The first geometric figure we will consider is the *rectangle*. It consists of four sides and four right angles (Fig. 4-12). In a rectangle the opposite sides are equal. Often the longer side is known as the length (l) and the shorter side as the width (w) or height (h).

The rectangle is a useful model with which to illustrate two properties of figures. One is the *perimeter;* it measures the length of the boundary around

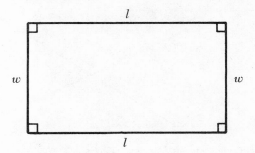

Fig. 4-12. A rectangle. All angles are 90 degrees.

the figure. For a rectangle of dimensions $l \times w$ the formula for the perimeter is $s = l + w + l + w = 2\,(l + w)$. Another property of the figure is the area. It measures the region within the boundary. The formula for the *area (A) of a rectangle* is as follows:

$$A = l \times w$$

Formula 4-3

Since the area is the product of two dimensions, it is expressed in units of length squared. Typical area units are square centimeters (cm^2) and square meters (m^2).

A flat body that exhibits perimeter and area but not thickness is called a "lamina." For practical purposes, thin sheets of uniform material, such as paper, x-ray film, plywood, or Lucite can be considered examples of laminae. To determine their masses (or weights) we use formula 4-3.

> **Example 4-5.** A certain x-ray film has a mass of 0.2 gm/cm². What is the mass of a piece of that film measuring 30 cm by 50 cm? The area is 30 × 50 = 1,500 cm²; the mass is 0.2 × 1,500 = 300 gm.

> **Example 4-6.** The wall of a diagnostic x-ray room is to be covered by lead foil giving protection of 3 gm/cm². If the wall is 10 m long and 3 m high, what is the weight of the foil? The dimensions of the wall are 1000 cm × 300 cm. The area is 1,000 × 300 = 300,000 cm². The mass is 3 × 300,000 = 900,000 gm, or 900 kg (0.9 metric tons).

> **Example 4-7.** A 9 × 9 inch floor tile is extracted from the floor of an isotope laboratory and analyzed. It is found to contain 0.1 μCi of contamination. Using this value as an approximate representation of the contamination on the floor, estimate the total contamination on a 10 × 12 foot floor. In other terms, 9 inches by 9 inches is 81 inches², or $^{81}/_{144}$ feet²; thus the contamination is 0.1/(81/144) $\cong$ 0.178 μCi/feet². The area of the floor is 10 × 12 = 120 ft². The comtamination estimate is 0.178 × 120 = 21 μCi.

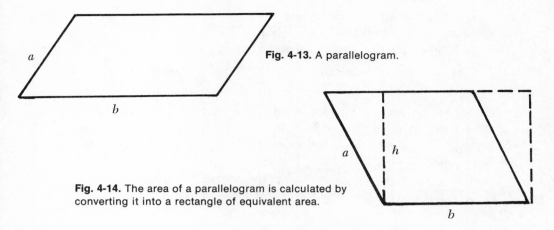

Fig. 4-13. A parallelogram.

Fig. 4-14. The area of a parallelogram is calculated by converting it into a rectangle of equivalent area.

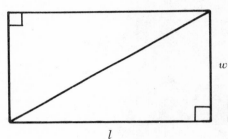

Fig. 4-15. A diagonal divides the rectangle into two right triangles.

The square and the parallelogram. A special type of rectangle is the *square*. It is simply a rectangle in which length and width are equal, in other words a closed figure with four equal sides and four right angles.

Another common four-sided figure is the *parallelogram,* an example of which is shown in Fig. 4-13. In it the opposite sides are parallel and have equal length. The perimeter of the parallelogram is the sum of the four sides. If two adjacent sides are labeled "a" and "b" (as in Fig. 4-13), the perimeter is $p = 2a + 2b = 2(a + b)$.

To compute the area of a parallelogram we convert it into a rectangle of equivalent area by removing a triangular portion from one end (Fig. 4-14) and moving it to the other end. The area of the parallelogram is seen to be the length of one side multiplied by the perpendicular distance to the opposite side (the height).

THE TRIANGLE AND THE CIRCLE. Of great importance in geometry—and the related trigonometry—is the *triangle*. Having only three sides, the triangle is the simplest straight-sided figure.* If one of its angles is a right angle, we speak of a *right triangle*. Any rectangle can be converted into a pair of equal right triangles by drawing a diagonal, as in Fig. 4-15. Conversely, if we add

---

*The triangle is a key item in engineering also. It is the only closed, straight-sided figure whose shape is determined by the length of its sides alone. This means that most triangular structures are naturally rigid.

to any triangle, not necessarily a right one, another equal triangle in the appropriate way, we obtain a parallelogram as in Fig. 4-16. It can be shown that the formula for the *area of a triangle* is as follows:

$$A = \tfrac{1}{2}bh$$

Formula 4-4

where b is the base (any side of the triangle) and h is the height (the perpendicular distance from the base to the opposite angle or vertex). The triangle will be used mainly for conceptual development of other aspects of geometry pertinent to radiology.

The final figure we will consider is the *circle*. It is a closed curved figure (Fig. 4-17). Three lengths are associated with a circle. The *radius* (r) is the distance from the center to any point on the rim or *circumference* (circumference is used in reference to circles only). The *diameter* (d) is the maximum distance across the circle, or twice the radius:

$$d = 2r$$

Formula 4-5

The perimeter or *length of the circumference* (C), is related to the radius or diameter by the following formula:

$$C = 2\pi r = \pi d$$

Formula 4-6

Here $\pi \cong 3.14$.

Example 4-8. To measure the magnification in radiographs a circle (loop) of radiopaque material of known size is placed near the object of interest. We wish to construct such a circle out of a single loop of lead wire. If the circle is to have a diameter of 5 cm, how long a wire do we need? The length needed is the circumference of a circle 5 cm in diameter, or length = 3.14 × 5 = 15.7 cm.

Example 4-9. A piece of lead foil is 20 cm long. If it is rolled into a cylinder two layers thick (Fig. 4-18), what is the radius of the cylinder? The cylinder will have a circumference of 10 cm, or $10 = 2\pi r$, or $r = 10/2\pi \cong 1.6$ cm.

The *area of the circle* (A) also involves π. The formula is as follows:

$$A = \pi r^2$$

Formula 4-7

Example 4-10. What is the area of a 9-inch image-intensifier tube? The 9 inches refers to the diameter of the tube; in general, if the radius, diameter, or circumference is not specified, the diameter (at least in North American usage) is implied. The radius is 4.5 inches; the area is $A = \pi r^2 = 3.14 \times 4.5 \times 4.5 = 63.6$ inches^2.

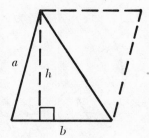

Fig. 4-16. A parallelogram can be obtained by adjoining two equal triangles. The area of the parallelogram is *bh;* thus, the area of one triangle must be ¹/₂ *bh.*

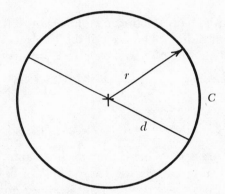

Fig. 4-17. The circle. The radius is *r*, diameter *d*, and circumference is *C*.

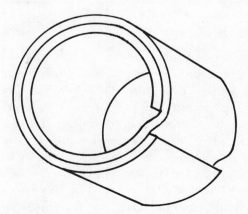

Fig. 4-18. A lead cylinder formed by rolling a rectangular sheet of lead.

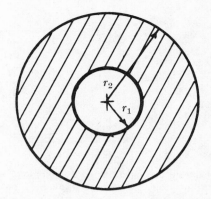

Fig. 4-19. An annulus. The annulus has an inner and an outer radius. The area of the annulus shown is the area of the circle with radius r_2 less the area of the circle with radius r_1, or $A = \pi(r_2^2 - r_1^2)$.

Example 4-11. What size square would have the same area as a circle 3 cm in radius? The area of the circle is equal to $3.14 \times 3 \times 3 = 28.3$ cm². The area of a square whose side is l is $l \times l$. Therefore:

$$l \times l = 28.3 \text{ cm}^2$$

or

$$l = \sqrt{28.3} \cong 5.3 \text{ cm}$$

Example 4-12. What is the area of an annulus (Fig. 4-19) of outer radius 10 cm and inner radius 3 cm? The area of the annulus is the area of the outer circle less the area of the inner circle. In this case:

$$\begin{aligned}
\text{Area} &= \pi 10^2 - \pi 3^2 \\
&= \pi(10^2 - 3^2) \cong 3.14(100 - 9) \\
&= 3.14 \times 91 = 286 \text{ cm}^2
\end{aligned}$$

GEOMETRIC THEOREMS

Geometry is often presented as a series of axioms, theorems, and corollaries. *Axioms* are unproved but obvious "truths"; an example is "any two distinct points determine a unique straight line." *Theorems* are major deductions based on axioms. Once proved, a theorem can be used to deduce further theorems. *Corollaries* are minor deductions from theorems. It is not our purpose to extensively develop the elegant edifice of the mathematics of geometry. However, a few theorems are so important that they will be briefly considered here. In some cases their proof will be incomplete.

CONGRUENT TRIANGLES. If two triangles are equal (in geometry they are called *congruent*), then the lengths of the corresponding sides of the triangles are equal. The converse is also true, that is, if all sides of one triangle are equal

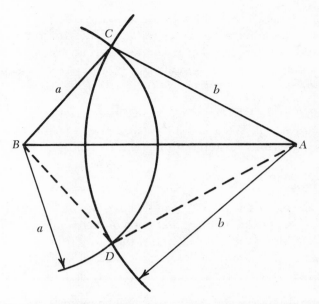

Fig. 4-20. Equal triangles. We can construct a triangle equal to triangle *ABC* by drawing one arc of radius *a* centered at *B* and a second arc of radius *b* centered at *A*. By joining the intersection of the two arcs *(D)* to the points *A* and *B,* we form a mirror image of the original triangle.

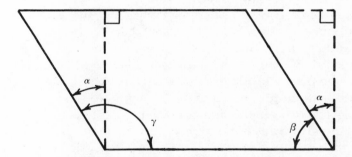

Fig. 4-21. A parallelogram converted to a rectangle of equal area by removing the right triangle shown on the left and placing it on the right. The two triangles are equal. The angle β is 90° − α and the angle γ is 90° + α; thus $\beta + \gamma$ is equal to 180 degrees.

to the corresponding sides of a second triangle, the two triangles are equal. This can be shown by constructing a triangle with sides equal to an existing triangle. The construction of a second triangle that shares one side as a common base is shown in Fig. 4-20.

If we add the measures of all the four angles in a rectangle, we obtain 360 degrees, since each angle is 90 degrees. For a parallelogram the situation is a little more complicated, but can be analyzed by the construct shown in Fig. 4-21. By adding α to a right angle on one side and subtracting α from a right angle on the other side, we can see that β and γ at the bottom of the parallelogram add up to 180 degrees. Thus in a parallelogram the four angles total 360 degrees, just as in a rectangle.

Probably even more important than the properties of a parallelogram are the properties of a triangle. As we saw before in Fig. 4-16, two equal triangles can be adjoined to form a parallelogram. Since these triangles are equal, they must have equal corresponding angles. This means that the 360 degrees of the parallelogram are shared equally by both triangles. This implies that *the sum of the three angles in a triangle is always 180 degrees*.

Example 4-13. A triangle contains one right angle; the other two angles are equal. What are the measures of these equal angles? Call these angles α. The sum of the angles in the triangle is $\alpha + \alpha + 90° = 180°$, or $2\alpha + 90° = 180°$; hence $\alpha = \dfrac{180° - 90°}{2} = 45°$.

Example 4-14. Can a triangle have two obtuse angles? An obtuse angle is greater than 90 degrees; two obtuse angles would add to more than 180 degrees, which is more than any triangle can have. Therefore a triangle cannot have two obtuse angles.

An important special case is the right triangle. A right triangle contains two acute angles; these angles must add to 90 degrees, that is, the two acute angles in a right triangle are complementary.

PYTHAGOREAN THEOREM. Another formula useful in many situations is the *Pythagorean theorem,* named for Pythagoras, the Greek mathematician who first discovered the relationship about 2,500 years ago. In right triangles it is conventional to call the long side, the side opposite the 90 degree angle, the *hypotenuse*. Four equal right triangles of base (b), height (h), and hypotenuse (r) can be placed inside two equal squares whose sides have a length of $b + h$. Two patterns for arranging the triangles are shown in Fig. 4-22. Since the areas of the two squares and of their internal triangles are equal, the areas of the internal squares not covered by the triangles must also be equal. In one case, the uncovered area is r^2, or the "square of the hypotenuse"; in the other case, the sum of the areas of the two small squares $b^2 + h^2$ is "the sum of the squares of the other two sides." Equating these areas gives the following:

$$r^2 = b^2 + h^2$$

Formula 4-8

or in words: *The square of the hypotenuse is equal to the sum of the squares of the two other sides*.

Example 4-15. A right triangle has a base of 4 cm and a height of 3 cm. How long is the hypotenuse? The Pythagorean theorem gives $r^2 = b^2 + h^2$, or $r^2 = 4^2 + 3^2 = 25$; hence $r = 5$ cm.

Example 4-16. How long is the diagonal of a square with sides of 1 cm? The diagonal of the square and two sides form a right triangle with the diagonal as the hypotenuse. The Pythagorean theorem gives $r^2 = 1^2 + 1^2$; or $r^2 = 1 + 1$; hence $r = \sqrt{2}$ (the square root of 2 is approximately 1.414, a number worth remembering).

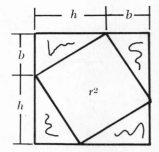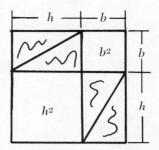

Fig. 4-22. The Pythagorean theorem. Four equal right triangles of base b and height h are laid inside two equal squares whose sides are $b + h$. In both cases the area left uncovered (r^2 and $b^2 + h^2$) must be equal. At left, r^2 is "the square of the hypotenuse"; at right $b^2 + h^2$ is "the sum of the squares of the other two sides."

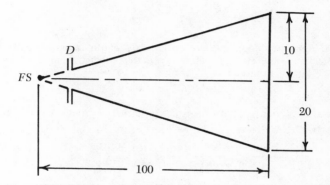

Fig. 4-23. An x-ray beam. At left, the focal spot *(FS)* and diaphragm *(D)* at right, a 20 cm cassette. The edge of the beam corresponds to the hypotenuse of a right triangle whose two other sides, in this case, are 10 and 100 cm long. Figure is not to scale.

Example 4-17. An x-ray beam is 20 cm wide when it strikes a cassette 100 cm from the focal point; more exactly, the distance from the focal point to the center of the cassette is 100 cm. This is illustrated in Fig. 4-23. How far is the edge of the field from the focal point? The edge of the beam and the cassette form a triangle; a bisector divides this triangle into two right triangles whose short sides are 100 cm and 10 cm. Application of the Pythagorean theorem shows that the hypotenuse of these right triangles is $\sqrt{100^2 + 10^2} = \sqrt{10{,}000 + 100} = \sqrt{10{,}100} \cong 100.5$ cm. This is the length we wished to find.

Example 4-18. An object whose length (l) is known to be 20 cm is viewed from point A (Fig. 4-24); it appears to be 10 cm long (l_A). How long will l_B appear when viewed from point B if the line from B to the object forms a right angle with the line from A to the object? (Points A and B and the object all lie in the same plane). The object l, and

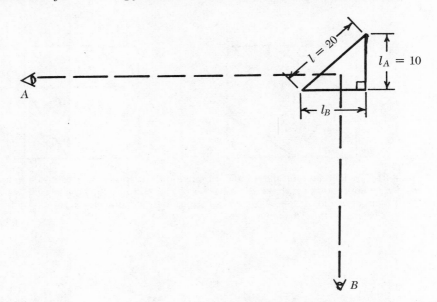

Fig. 4-24. View of an angulated object. The true length *l* and the apparent lengths l_A and l_B are related by the formula $l^2 = l_A{}^2 + l_B{}^2$. Note that the object must be in the same plane as the points *A* and *B*. Figure is not to scale.

---

the two apparent lengths l_A and l_B form a right triangle, with *l* being the hypotenuse. The lengths obey the condition $l^2 = l_A{}^2 + l_B{}^2$. This can be solved for l_B: $l_B = \sqrt{l^2 - l_A{}^2}$, or, numerically, $l_B = \sqrt{20^2 - 10^2} = \sqrt{400 - 100} \cong 17.32$.

Two special right triangles whose angles can be related to the ratio of the side lengths can be developed. An *equilateral* triangle is one in which all the sides are of equal length. Such a triangle (*ABD* is shown in Fig. 4-25). All angles in an equilateral triangle are equal; this means that each is $^{180°}/_3 = 60°$. A line from the apex to the middle of the base divides the apex angle in half and forms a right angle with the base. Thus this bisector, half the base, and one full side enclose a right triangle (*ABC* in Fig. 4-25). Such a triangle is often called a "30-60-90" triangle in reference to the angles. Its hypotenuse is *l* and the base is $^1/_2$. Its third side, the height, is found by the equation $l^2 = (^1/_2)^2 + h^2$, or $h^2 = l^2 - \dfrac{l^2}{4} = (^3/_4)l^2$, or $h = l\sqrt{^3/_4} = l\dfrac{\sqrt{3}}{2}$.

The ratio of base to hypotenuse is $\dfrac{^1/_2}{l} = {}^1/_2$, the ratio of height to hypotenuse of *l* is $\dfrac{l\sqrt{^3/_2}}{l} = \dfrac{\sqrt{3}}{2}$ (about 0.866), and the ratio of height to base is $\dfrac{l\sqrt{^3/_2}}{l/2} = \sqrt{3}$. By calling $l = 2$ we can express a ratio of hypotenuse to height to base as $2:\sqrt{3}:1$. These ratios are true for all 30-60-90 triangles.

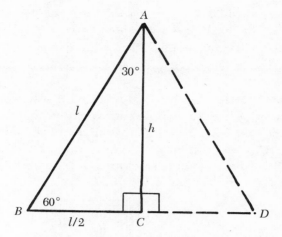

Fig. 4-25. Two right triangles with angles of 30°, 60°, and 90° obtained by cutting the equilateral triangle *ABD* in half.

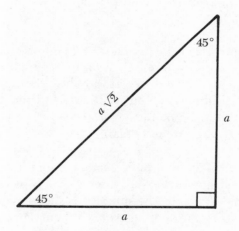

Fig. 4-26. A 45°- 45°- 90° triangle.

Example 4-19. The height of a 30-60-90 triangle is 20 cm. How long is the base? Call the height h and the base b. The ratio h/b is equal to $\sqrt{3}/1$ (since this is a 30-60-90 triangle), and $b = h/\sqrt{3} \cong 11.6$.

Note that Fig. 4-24 represents a 30-60-90 triangle.

Another important right triangle is the one with two equal sides shown in Fig. 4-26. The two acute angles must be 45 degrees, since they are equal. Thus we can call this a 45-45-90 triangle. If the length of a short side is a, the hypotenuse must be $\sqrt{a^2 + a^2} = \sqrt{2a^2} = a\sqrt{2}$ and the ratios of the sides are $\sqrt{2}:1:1$.

Example 4-20. How long is the diagonal of a square with 25 cm sides? The diagonal and two sides form a 45-45-90 triangle with the diagonal as hypotenuse. Thus the diagonal is $25\sqrt{2}$ cm ($\cong 35.4$ cm).

SIMILAR TRIANGLES. Our final theorem involves *similar triangles*. They can be defined as triangles whose corresponding angles are equal. An example is shown in Fig. 4-27. Notice that similar triangles usually do not have the same size. (Obviously, if they do, they are congruent.) If corresponding sides are identified (corresponding sides are opposite the equal angles), their ratios are equal. For the example in Fig. 4-27:

$$\frac{a}{A} = \frac{b}{B} = \frac{c}{C}$$

Formula 4-9

This theorem is: *The ratio of the corresponding sides of similar triangles is constant;* for the particular example of Fig. 4-27 the constant is 2. This theorem can be shown to apply readily to similar 30-60-90 triangles or 45-45-90 triangles.

Example 4-21. The hypotenuse of one 30-60-90 triangle is three times the hypotenuse of another similar triangle. Show, without using the last theorem, that the corresponding shortest sides are in the ratio of 3 to 1. Call the hypotenuses $3L$ and L respectively. The short sides are one half the hypotenuse in a 30-60-90 triangle. They are $^{3L}/_2$ and $^{L}/_2$; the ratio between them is plainly 3 to 1.

Example 4-22. A pinhole camera is set up with the pinhole 20 cm from the focal spot of an x-ray tube. A film is placed at 80 cm from the focal spot and exposed. The situation is shown in Fig. 4-28. When the film is developed, the spot measures 1.2 cm. How big is the focal spot? Provided the focal spot is parallel to the film, the triangle to the left of the diaphragm is similar to the triangle to the right. Since the height of the triangle to the left is one third of the triangle to the right, the focal spot is one third of the size of the image on the film, or $\dfrac{1.2}{3} = 0.4$ cm.

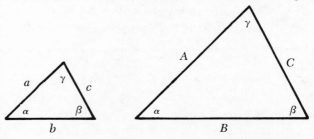

Fig. 4-27. Similar triangles. The sides of the larger triangle are twice as long as the corresponding sides of the smaller one, but their corresponding angles are equal.

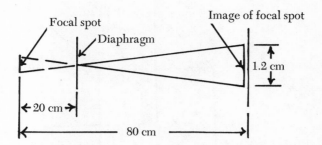

Focal spot
Diaphragm
Image of focal spot
1.2 cm
20 cm
80 cm

Fig. 4-28. Pinhole camera image of the focal spot of an x-ray tube. The triangles to the left and right of the diaphragm are similar; their heights measure 20 and 60 cm, respectively.

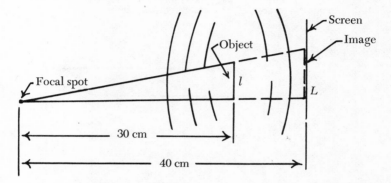

Screen
Image
Object
Focal spot
l
L
30 cm
40 cm

Fig. 4-29. The x-ray magnification of an object projected on a screen.

Example 4-23. An object is viewed on a fluoroscope having a distance of 40 cm between focal spot and screen. What is the magnification if the object is 10 cm in front of the screen? This is shown in Fig. 4-29. If the object's length is l and image L, the magnification is L/l. The triangle with solid lines and the one with the extended dotted lines are similar and their ratio is 3 to 4; thus L/l is $4/3$ or 1.33. This is the magnification for this object. Notice that the magnification varies for objects that are at varying distances from the screen.

THREE-DIMENSIONAL FIGURES

THE CUBE AND RECTANGULAR PARALLELEPIPED. A three-dimensional figure in which all angles are 90 degrees and all sides are equal is called a *cube*. An example is shown in Fig. 4-30. Another three-dimensional figure is the *rectangular parallelepiped* shown in Fig. 4-31.

The volume of a solid object tells us how much material it contains. The inside volume of a container indicates its carrying capacity. The volume of an object can be thought of as the amount of liquid a container of the same inside shape can hold. It can be measured in liters, quarts, gallons, or units of the

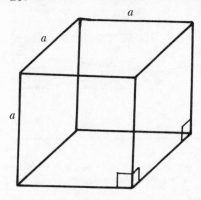

Fig. 4-30. A cube. All angles are 90 degrees, and all sides have the same length, *a*. Each of the six sides is a square of area a^2. The volume of the cube is a^3.

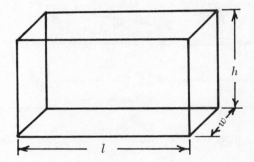

Fig. 4-31. A rectangular parallelepiped. Each side is a rectangle, and all angles are 90 degrees. The volume is $l \times w \times h$.

cube of length. The volume of a cube with sides of 1 cm is 1 cm³; it is equal to 1 milliliter (ml).

> **Example 4-24.** How many liters are there in a cube 1 m on a side? Each meter is 100 cm. Thus the volume 1 m³ = 100 × 100 × 100 = 10^6 cm³ and 1 cm³ = 1 × 10^{-3} liters (since 1 cm³ contains 1 ml). Combining these, 1 m³ = 10^6 cm³ = 10^6 × 10^{-3} = 10^3 liters.

The liter is a convenient measurement for everyday activities such as buying gasoline or milk. The cubic centimeter or the milliliter is more convenient for laboratory use.

> **Example 4-25.** A standard lead brick is approximately 5 × 10 × 20 cm. What is the volume? It is 5 × 10 × 20 = 1,000 cm³ (or 1 liter or 10^{-3} m³).

SOME COMMON DENSITIES

Air	1.3×10^{-3} gm/cm^3
Water	1 gm/cm^3
Aluminum	2.7 gm/cm^3
Lead	11.3 gm/cm^3
Mercury	13.5 gm/cm^3

Example 4-26. How long should a side of a cube be so that its volume will be 1,000 cm^3? If we call the side length a, then $a \times a \times a = a^3 = 1,000$, or $a = \sqrt[3]{1,000} = 10$ cm.

Example 4-27. The bottom of a water phantom is 30 × 40 cm. How many liters of water will be required to fill it to a depth of 15 cm? The volume of the water will be $30 \times 40 \times 15 = 18,000$ cm^3, or 18 liters.

An important aspect of the volume is its mass density; this is usually just called *density* and is often designated by the Greek letter ρ (rho). The mass M, the volume V, and the density are related by the following formula:

$$\rho = {}^M\!/_V \qquad\qquad \textbf{Formula 4-10}$$

For most homogeneous materials ρ is constant or nearly so. A few typical values are shown in the boxed material on this page.

Example 4-28. What is the mass of 1 liter of mercury? Since 1 liter is 10^3 cm^3 and the density is = 13.5 gm/cm^3, the mass will be 13.5×10^3 = 13,500 gm, or 13.5 kg (about 30 pounds).

Example 4-29. How many kilograms of lead are needed to cover a wall with 2 mm of foil if the wall is 3 m high and 5 wide? Changing the dimensions to centimeters, the sizes are 0.2 × 300 × 500; the volume is 30,000 cm^3. The mass is $11.3 \times 30,000 = 339,000$ gm, or 339 kg (about $^1/_3$ metric ton).

Example 4-30. A 5 kg roll of lead foil is 0.5 m wide and the foil is 0.2 mm thick. How long is the roll? The volume (in cubic centimeters) is $0.02 \times 50 \times L = 1 \times L$ where L is the length. The mass is $1 \times L \times 11.3$ = 5,000 gm; $L = 442$ cm, or 4.42 m.

In evaluating physical problems it is important to use a "consistent" set of units. To add 2 m to 10 cm, we must convert one value to the units of the other or both to another unit. Throughout our examples in this portion, we will use centimeters for length and grams for mass. Except for certain engineering applications, such as the measurement of shielding, these are commonly used units. No explicit examples using nonmetric values are given. For conversion, 1 inch ≅ 2.54 cm (or approximately 4 inches = 10 cm), 1 pound ≅ 454 gm (or approximately 2 pounds = 1 kg), and 1 U.S. quart ≅ 0.9 liters.

THE CYLINDER. For a rectangular parallelepiped the formula for determining volume is length × width × height. It can be seen that this is equivalent to the area of the base × the height, since the area of the base is determined by the length × the width. This relationship:

$$V = A \times h$$

Formula 4-11

is *true for all bodies that maintain the same horizontal cross-sectional area at all levels*. If the figure is tilted, h is the vertical height. This is illustrated for a tilted cylinder in Fig. 4-32. For a *right circular cylinder* of radius r and length l, as shown in Fig. 4-33, the area of one end is πr^2; thus the volume is as follows:

$$V = \pi r^2 l$$

Formula 4-12

The volumes of cylindrical prisms with cross sections of a parallelogram or a triangle can also be found by formula 4-11.

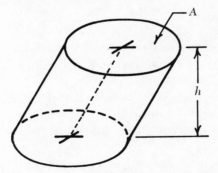

Fig. 4-32. A tilted cylinder. The volume of the cylinder is the area of the base *(A)* multiplied by the perpendicular distance *(h)* between the ends. A cylinder has the same cross section throughout its length *(h)*.

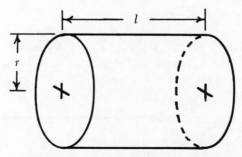

Fig. 4-33. A right circular cylinder. The volume is $\pi r^2 l$. The area of each end is πr^2, and the curved side is $2\pi r l$. The total surface area is $2\pi r^2 + 2\pi r l$ or $2\pi r \, (r + l)$.

Example 4-31. What is the volume of a ^{60}Co source that is in the shape of a cylinder 2 cm in diameter and 2 cm long? The radius is 1 cm. Using formula 4-12 the volume is $\pi \times 1^2 \times 2 = \pi \times 2 = 6.28$ cm³.

Example 4-32. How many liters of radioactive waste will a drum 1 m high and 30 cm in radius hold? The volume will be $\pi \times 30^2 \times 100 = 2.83 \times 10^5$ cm³, or 283 liters.

Example 4-33. A waste container is needed with a volume of at least 7,000 cm³. It is to be made by stacking round lead rings of 20 cm inside diameter and 5 cm high. The problem is illustrated in Fig. 4-34. What is the minimum number of rings needed? Each ring holds a volume of $\pi \times 10^2 \times 5 = 1,571$ cm³. The number of rings must be $\dfrac{7,000}{1,571} = 4.46$. If only full-height rings can be used, a total of 5 is the minimum needed.

Example 4-34. The outer diameter of the rings in the preceding example is 30 cm. What is the volume of lead in the stack of 5 rings? The cross section of a ring is an annulus with an inside radius of 10 cm and an outside radius of 15 cm. Its area is $\pi(15^2 - 10^2) = 393$ cm². The volume of 1 ring is $5 \times 393 = 1,964$ cm³ and of 5 rings about 9,820 cm³.

Example 4-35. How many liters of solution will be held by a bucket approximately 30 cm in diameter and 25 cm high? The volume is $\pi r^2 h \cong 3.14 \times 15^2 \times 25 = 1.77 \times 10^4$ cm³, or 17.7 liters.

The surface area of a cylinder is the sum of the areas at each end and of the curved side. The area at one end of a right circular cylinder (Fig. 4-33) is πr^2. The curved surface can be thought of as a rectangle that has been "rolled up" into a pipe. This rectangle has one side equal to the perimeter ($2\pi r$) of the

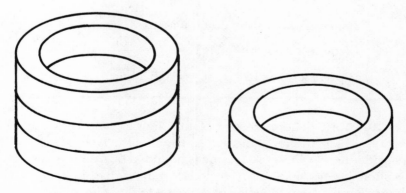

Fig. 4-34. A cylindrical shield made from lead rings. The usable space inside the shield is a right circular cylinder. The base of the shield is an annulus. The volume of lead is the area of the annulus multiplied by the height.

circle; the other dimension is the height (h) of the cylinder. Thus the total area is $\pi r^2 + \pi r^2 + 2\pi rh$, that is, the *surface area of a right circular cylinder* is as follows:

$$A = 2\pi r(r + h)$$

Formula 4-13

Example 4-36. A shield for xenon bags has the form of a cylinder 40 cm in diameter and 50 cm long. How many square centimeters of lead foil are needed to make this shield? The area needed is $2\pi r(r + h) = 2 \times 3.14 \times 20 \times (20 + 50) = 8.8 \times 10^3$ cm².

Another three-dimensional figure is the *sphere*. For this figure the volume is as follows:

$$V = \frac{4\pi r^3}{3}$$

Formula 4-14

and the surface area is:

$$A = 4\pi r^2$$

Formula 4-15

The derivations of these formulas will not be given here.

Example 4-37. A certain droplet of liquid is 1 mm (0.1 cm) across. What is its volume? The volume is $4 \times 3.14 \times 0.05^3/3 = 5.2 \times 10^{-4}$ cm³.

Example 4-38. It takes about ten drops of water from an eyedropper to make 1 cm³. What is the diameter of these drops? The volume (V) is 0.1 cm³. Since $V = \dfrac{4\pi r^3}{3}$, $r = \sqrt[3]{\dfrac{3V}{4\pi}} = \sqrt[3]{0.0239} \cong 0.29$ cm and the diameter is 0.58 cm.

Example 4-39. How much mass is in a piece of lead shot 1.5 mm in diameter? The volume is $V = \dfrac{4\pi(0.075)^3}{3} = 1.77 \times 10^{-3}$ cm³. The mass is $\rho V = 11.3 \times 1.77 \times 10^{-3} = 0.020$ gm.

THE CONE. There are many other figures whose formula for volume or area can be found in mathematical handbooks. The only other figure we will consider here is the *cone*. A cone is bounded by a flat surface, the *base* (which is often, but not necessarily, a circle), and a surface defined by all the straight lines running from the *apex* of the cone to the edge of the base. A cone with a semicircular base is shown in Fig. 4-35. *For any cone* the volume is given as follows:

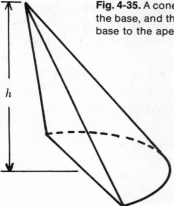

Fig. 4-35. A cone with a semicircular base. A cone is bounded by a flat surface, the base, and the surfaces made by the lines drawn from the boundary of the base to the apex.

h

FS

50

10

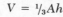

10

Fig. 4-36. A shaped block (heavy lines). It is part of a cone formed by a beam emanating from a focal spot *(FS)*.

$$V = \tfrac{1}{3}Ah$$

Formula 4-16

A is the area of the base and h the vertical height from base to apex.

Example 4-40. If the radius of the semicircular base in Fig. 4-35 is 10 cm and the vertical height is 15 cm, what is the volume? The area of the base is that of half a circle, or $\tfrac{1}{2}\pi r^2$; $V = \tfrac{1}{3}Ah = \tfrac{1}{3}(\tfrac{1}{2}\pi r^2)h = \tfrac{1}{3}(\tfrac{1}{2} \times 3.14 \times 10^2) \times 15 = 785$ cm^3.

Example 4-41. Fig. 4-36 illustrates a shaped block whose edges are parallel to a beam emanating from a focal spot. Because the beam diverges, the block appears as part of a cone. If the bottom of the block measures 10×10 cm and is 50 cm from the source or focal spot and the block is 10 cm high, what is its volume? The volume of the block is the difference between the volume of the cone with its base at the bottom of the block and the volume of the cone with its base at the top of the block. In both cases the apex of the cone is the focal spot. By using similar triangles the top of the block can be shown to be 8×8 cm. The volume of the larger cone is $\frac{1}{3}Ah = \frac{1}{3} \times 10^2 \times 50 = 1{,}667$ cm^3 and the smaller is $\frac{1}{3} \times 8^2 \times 40 = 853$ cm^3. Thus the volume of the shaped block is $1{,}667 - 853 = 814$ cm^3.

PROJECTIVE GEOMETRY

Of great importance is the evaluation of magnified objects. Magnification and its relationship to the relative position of object and image to the focal spot are illustrated in Fig. 4-29. The role of the distances between source, object, and image was discussed in that connection. Here we will be concerned with the study of area and volume as modified by magnification. This magnification can be a real modification of the appearance of an object or it can simply be a uniform scaling. An example of uniform scaling is shown in Fig. 4-27, where the sides of one triangle are exactly twice as long as the corresponding sides in the other triangle. Image magnification can be achieved by such means as a diverging beam (as in Fig. 4-29), a camera (Fig. 4-28), or optical lenses.

LINEAR PROJECTION. First, we will consider the case of linear projection where we have a collimated beam originating from a point source as shown in Fig. 4-37. To the right of the aperture the beam width is an image of the collimators. That is, the object is the collimator width (w) and is situated at a distance (l) from the source. At other distances the beam width and the source form a triangle similar to that formed by the source and the object. Thus the width of the beam at $2l$ from the source is exactly twice the width of the object.

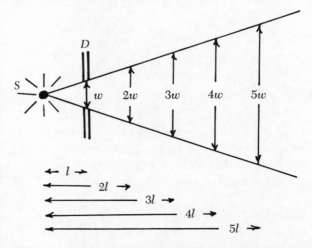

Fig. 4-37. A collimated beam. The width of the beam is directly proportional to the distance from the source *S* (not the collimator, *D*). For example, at 4*l* the beam is twice as wide as it is at 2*l*.

At a distance of $3l$ the width is $3w$ and so on. It can be seen that the beam width is directly proportional to the distance from the source, often called r.

> **Example 4-42.** An x-ray beam is 20 cm wide at the cassette, which is 100 cm from the focal spot (as in Fig. 4-23). If the collimators are 20 cm from the focal spot, how far apart are they? Call the separation of the collimators d. Then $d/_{20} = {}^{20}/_{100}$; solving for d shows that d is 4 cm.

> **Example 4-43.** How wide is the beam of the preceding example at 80 cm from the focal spot? Call this width w; then $w/_{80} = {}^{20}/_{100}$, or $w = 16$ cm.

AREA AND VOLUME PROJECTION. When a beam of square or rectangular cross section is considered, each side of the square increases proportional to the distance (r). The area is the product of two sides. For example, if the distance from the source is doubled, the beam width and depth are doubled and the area is increased by a factor of $4 (= 2^2)$. This can be seen in Fig. 4-38.

In Fig. 4-39 the projection of a round figure is shown. Here the radius increases linearly with the distance. Since the area obeys formula 4-7 $(A = \pi r^2)$, the area of this beam increases as the square of the distance.

In general, whether the projected area is a regular figure or not, the area will increase as the square of the distance from a point source increases. Furthermore, even if a point source is not identified, as long as the linear dimensions are all scaled by a uniform factor (f), the area increases by f^2. An example of this is Fig. 4-27, in which the linear dimensions are increased by a factor of 2. The area increases by a factor of 4.

> **Example 4-44.** An x-ray beam is 8×8 cm where it enters a patient 80 cm from the focal spot. What is the area of this beam at the patient's midline 10 cm beyond the entry point? The field edges are

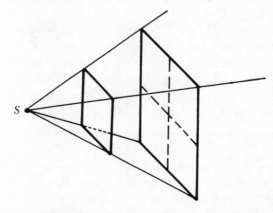

Fig. 4-38. Area projection. If the distance from the source *(S)* is doubled, as in this case, the area will increase four times.

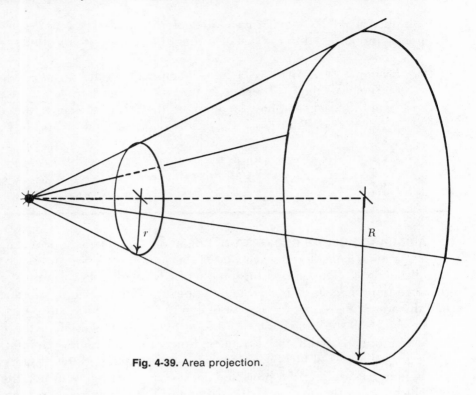

Fig. 4-39. Area projection.

$8 \times {}^{90}/_{80} = 9$ cm long. The area is 9×9. Or, the area on the skin is $8 \times 8 = 64$ cm². The area at 10 cm depth is $64 \times ({}^{90}/_{80})^2 = 81$ cm².

Example 4-45. The liver on a ¼-scale photograph of a scan appears to have an area of 15 cm². What would the area have been if the photograph were life size? The area is proportional to the square of the size; therefore the area in the life-size scan should be $4^2 = 16$ times the area of the small photograph. The full size area is $15 \times 16 = 240$ cm².

Example 4-46. The dosage for a certain drug is proportional to the area of the skin. If 100 "units" are to be given to a six-foot (183 cm) individual of normal weight, what dosage should be given to a four-foot (112 cm) child of normal weight? The heights are in the ratio of 4 to 6 or ²/₃. The skin areas will be in the ratio of $(^2/_3)^2 = 0.44$. The dosage should be $0.44 \times 100 = 44$ "units."

Occasionally we are interested in the scaling of volume. If we have a cube of length l on a side, the volume is l^3. Thus the volume of a cube scales as the cube of the linear dimension. If a sphere is considered, the volume is given by formula 4-14: $V = \dfrac{4\pi r^3}{3}$. If the radius increases, the volume will increase as the cube of the radius. In general, the volume of a scaled object is related to the cube of the linear dimension.

> **Example 4-47.** In a half-size anatomical model, a certain organ has a volume of 5.2 cm³. What is the volume at full size? The full-size volume is $2^3 = 8$ times the half-size volume; it is $8 \times 5.2 = 41.6$ cm³.

> **Example 4-48.** Two individuals have similar builds. If one is 11% taller than the other, estimate the difference in weight. The weight or mass is proportional to the volume. The linear dimension of the larger individual is 1.11 times the linear dimension of the other. The volume, or mass, of the larger individual should be about $(1.11)^3 = 1.37$ times the volume or mass of the smaller. Thus we estimate the weight of the taller to be 37% more.

INVERSE SQUARE AND SOLID ANGLE

Many radiation problems assume the following conditions:
1. The radiation source is a "point" source.
2. The radiation is emitted equally in all directions.
3. The radiation travels in a straight line.
4. There is no significant absorption of the radiation.

These conditions also apply to small light sources such as ordinary light bulbs (particularly the unfrosted type).

INVERSE SQUARE. Under the conditions outlined the same radiation that passes through a small area nearby will also pass through the larger projected area farther away (Fig. 4-40).

If a *unit area* (for example, 1 cm²) is oriented at right angles to the radiation, the average amount of radiation that passes through the area in one second is the *flux* of radiation. If we wait for the entire procedure, the amount that has crossed the unit area is called the *fluence*. The amount of radiation can be measured in several ways. The most generally applicable are the number of particles and the energy. The number of particles gives the flux in particles per square centimeter-seconds (/cm²-sec) and the fluence in particles per

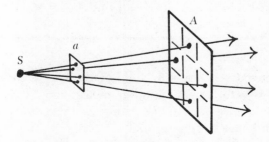

Fig. 4-40. Radiation from a point source *(S)*. As the radiation travels farther from the source, it spreads over a larger projected area. This reduces the intensity because the same amount of radiation has to cover more territory.

square centimeter. If the area is A and the time of observation is T, we have the following formulas:

$$Particle\ flux\ =\ \frac{Number\ of\ particles}{A \times T} \qquad \text{Formula 4-17}$$

$$Particle\ fluence\ =\ \frac{Number\ of\ particles}{A} \qquad \text{Formula 4-18}$$

Often the particle flux is given the symbol ϕ (Greek letter phi) and the fluence, Φ (capital phi). Comparing formulas 4-17 and 4-18 we see that:

$$\phi\ =\ \Phi/_T \qquad \text{Formula 4-19}$$

When the radiation is measured as energy used, fluence is energy per unit area and flux is energy per unit area-second. According to the International System of Units the energy is given in joules and the distance in meters. Thus fluence is expressed in joules per meter^2 (J/m^2) and flux as joules per meter^2-sec (J/m^2-sec) or watts per meter^2 (W/m^2). However, energy is often expressed in other units, such as ergs or electron volts, and the length in centimeters or smaller units. *Energy fluence* is given the symbol F and *energy flux, I*. The latter is also known as *intensity*.

> **Example 4-49.** Every second, 10,000 photons cross a square area 2 cm on a side. What is the flux? The area is $2 \times 2 = 4$ cm^2. The flux is $\frac{10,000}{4} = 2,500/$cm^2-sec.

> **Example 4-50.** If the flux of the preceding example continues for 5 seconds, what is the photon fluence? The fluence is $2,500 \times 5 = 12,500/$cm^2.

> **Example 4-51.** In a procedure lasting $1/10$ second, the energy fluence is $1/2$ J/m^2. What was the average energy flux during that time? The flux is $I = \dfrac{1/2}{1/10} = 1/2 \times 10 = 5$ J/m^2-sec.

Two specialized radiation fields will also be considered. For photons of energy 10 keV to 3 meV, another measure of fluence is the *exposure* (X), measured in *roentgens* (R). The exposure is directly proportional to the photon fluence, but is not so simply related to energy. A convenient measure of light intensity is the *luminous flux* measured in *lumens per square meter*. Because the sensitivity of the eye is involved, the luminous flux can only be related to the energy or photon flux if the color distribution or spectrum is known.

A very important aspect of fluence and flux is that they represent an amount of radiation traversing a unit area. Radiation from a point source will spread in many directions. The same radiation from a point source that passes through an area a at distance r in Fig. 4-40 will pass through an area $A\,(^R/_r)^2$ at distance R. Since the projected area increases as the square of the distance, the flux must decrease in proportion. Thus if the flux is $\phi(r)$ at a distance r, then the flux at a distance R is $\phi(R) = \phi(r) \times \left(\dfrac{r}{R}\right)^2$; if the flux at unit distance is ϕ_o, then at any other distance (r) it is as follows:

$$\phi(r) = \phi_0/r^2 \hspace{3cm} \text{Formula 4-20}$$

This is the very important *inverse square law*. It holds for all fluences and fluxes from a radiation source that meet the conditions outlined in the first paragraph of this section.

> **Example 4-52.** At 1 m from a light bulb the luminous flux is 10 lumens/m². What is the luminous flux at 2 m? Using formula 4-20, we see that the luminous flux is $^{10}/_{2^2} = 2.5$ lumens/m² at 2 m.

> **Example 4-53.** HEW rules require that light localizers for radiographic equipment must "provide an average *illumination* of not less than 160 *lux** at 100 cm or at the maximum source-image receptor distance (SID) whichever is less." Suppose a radiographic system is to be modified so that the SID will increase from 60 to 80 cm. If the light system at 60 cm just meets the requirement, how much brighter must the new light be? With the old light the illumination at 80 cm would be $160 \times (^{60}/_{80})^2 = 160(0.75)^2 = 160 \times .562 = 90$ lux. The illumination must be increased by a factor of $^{160}/_{90} = 1.78$ to meet the requirement.

> **Example 4-54.** At 1 cm from a radium point source of 1 mCi covered by 0.5 mm of platinum, the exposure is $X = 8.25$ R/hr. What is the exposure at 1 m from such a source? The exposure is $X = 8.25 \div (100)^2 = 8.25 \times 10^{-4}$ R/hr, or 0.825 mR/hr.

SOLID ANGLE. A common problem is the translation of output in, for example, particles per second, to the appropriate flux at a certain distance. Consider a point source emitting 3.7×10^7 photons/sec (this might be a 1 mCi source emitting one photon per decay); we want to know the particle flux 1 cm from this source. The emitted particles are equally likely to go in any direction. What is the chance that a particle will go through our defined unit area at a unit distance $(r = 1 \text{ cm})$ from the source (Fig. 4-41)? The surface area of a unit sphere is $A = 4\pi r^2 = 4\pi 1^2 = 4\pi \cong 12.56$ cm². The unit area measures 1

---

*One lux is the illumination produced by 1 lumen/m².

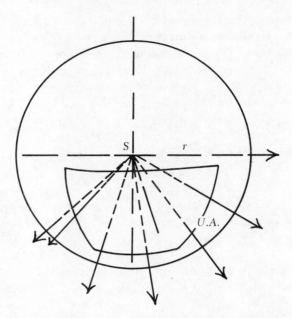

Fig. 4-41. Unit sphere and unit area on its surface. A point source *(S)* of radiation situated at the center of an imaginary sphere of 1 cm radius *(r)*. One square centimeter of the sphere surface is occupied by a unit area *(UA)*, which serves to measure the radiation flux and fluence.

cm². Thus the chance of its passing through the unit area is $\frac{1}{4\pi} \cong 0.080$. For our source emitting $3.7 = 10^7$ photons each second, the flux at 1 cm from the source is $3.7 \times \frac{10^7}{4\pi} = 2.9 \times 10^6$ photons/cm². This illustrates an important formula for translating output into flux or fluence:

$$Fluence\ at\ unit\ distance\ =\ Output/4\pi \qquad \text{\textbf{Formula 4-21}}$$

The flux is simply fluence per unit time.

> **Example 4-55.** Find the intensity in joules per square meter per second for a source of energy emitting 300 J/sec. Since the length is given in terms of meters, the unit distance is 1 m. The energy flux or intensity is $300/4\pi = 23.9$ J/m²-sec at 1 m from the source.

The procedure just used can be formalized by the use of the *solid angle*. This is an important concept for the determination both of flux and of detector efficiency.

Before proceeding to the definition of the solid angle, a brief return will be made to a plane angle. If an object is viewed from a point, it *subtends* an angle at that point. The angle *subtended* depends on the object and the position of

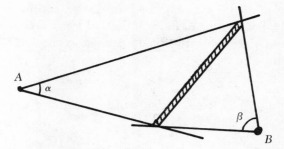

Fig. 4-42. Subtended angle. When viewed from point A the object subtends angle α. When viewed from position B the angle subtended is β.

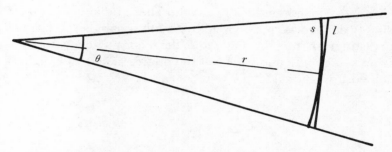

Fig. 4-43. The subtended angle. For objects at a distance much greater than their length, the subtended angle is approximately (in radians) the length divided by the distance. The subtended angle θ is exactly s/r; it is approximately l/r.

the point (Fig. 4-42). Specifically, the angle subtended depends on the length of the object, its angular orientation, and the distance. An object subtends a larger angle as its length increases, its orientation approaches 90 degrees, or it is moved closer. If viewed at right angles at a distance r, a small straight object of length l will subtend an angle $\theta \cong l/r$ (Fig. 4-43).

> **Example 4-56.** What is the approximate angle subtended at the focal spot by a 20 cm wide field at a distance of 100 cm? (This is the situation in Fig. 4-23.) The angle is approximately $^{20}/_{100} = 0.2$ radian (or $0.2 \times \dfrac{180}{\pi} = 11.5°$).

> **Example 4-57.** What is the angle subtended at the pinhole by the focal spot in Fig. 4-28? It is equal to the angle subtended by the image, or $\theta = \dfrac{1.2}{60} = 0.02$ radian, or $1.1°$.

Almost all useful radiation beams exhibit not just one dimension, a beam width, but a beam area, or field. If the field has a rectangular shape ($l \times w$ at distance r in Fig. 4-44), the beam can be expressed by the two angles subtended at the source.

$$\theta_1 \cong {}^l/_r \quad \text{and} \quad \theta_2 \cong {}^w/_r$$

A combined form, with θ_1 and θ_2 still in radians, gives the solid angle:

$$\Omega = \theta_1 \times \theta_2 \cong \frac{lw}{r^2}$$

The capital Greek omega is a convenient single measure of the size of the field. The product lw is the area A of the field at a distance r. This formula leads to a convenient definition of the *solid angle:*

$$\Omega = \frac{A}{r^2} \qquad \qquad \text{Formula 4-22}$$

The area A need not be a rectangle. The solid angle has no true units, being simply defined as area divided by length squared. The word *steradian* is used to distinguish the solid angle from the plane angle measured in radians. There is no solid angle equivalent of the degree. The solid angle is usually represented by a capital Greek letter.

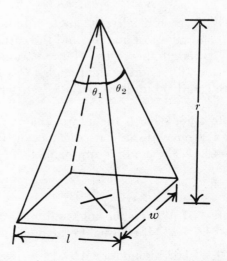

Fig. 4-44. Solid angle. It is the angular spread in two dimensions at the vertex of a cone. The size of the solid angle is determined by the area of the base ($l \times w$) and the height (r) of the cone.

If formula 4-22 is to be exact, the area (A) must be measured on the inner surface of a sphere of radius r centered at the vertex. For a complete spherical shell, the area is $4\pi r^2$. This shows that the maximum solid angle is 4π steradians.

If we return to the flux problem, we see that the radiation fraction (f) of an isotropic source (isotropic means radiating equally in all directions) that is contained in the solid angle Ω is as follows:

$$f = \Omega/4\pi \qquad \text{Formula 4-23}$$

Example 4-58. Find the solid angle subtended at the source by a square thermoluminescent dosimeter (TLD) chip of 0.2 cm side 50 cm from the source. The solid angle is given by formula 4-22 as $\dfrac{0.2 \times 0.2}{50 \times 50} = 1.6 \times 10^{-5}$ steradian.

Example 4-59. If the source in example 4-58 emits $N = 10^{10}$ particles, what is the number of particles that will strike the chip? The probability of any particle striking the chip is f of formula 4-23; the average number that strike the chip is $N \times f$. We find that f is $\dfrac{1.6 \times 10^{-5}}{4\pi}$ $\cong 1.27 \times 10^{-6}$, and that the number of particles that strike the chip is $1.27 \times 10^{-6} \times 10^{10} = 1.27 \times 10^{4}$.

Example 4-60. The area of the human pupil at its largest size is about 0.5 cm². What is the solid angle subtended by the pupil at a point 1 m from the eye? The solid angle is $\Omega = \dfrac{0.5}{100^2} = 5 \times 10^{-5}$ steradian.

Example 4-61. Use the results of the previous example to find the number of photons that enter the eye each second from a source 1 m away emitting 10^8 photons/sec. The number will be $\dfrac{5 \times 10^{-5}}{4\pi} \times 10^8 \cong 4.0 \times 10^2$ photons/sec.

CHAPTER REVIEW

1. What is an angle? A right angle? A negative angle?
2. How many degrees are there in a right angle? A full revolution?
3. What are the common properties of a square and a rectangle? What properties differentiate them?
4. Define the perimeter of a rectangle; What is the formula for the perimeter?
5. What is the formula for the area of a triangle? For the area of a circle?
6. When two lines intersect, what is the relationship between adjacent angles and opposite angles?
7. What is the relationship between angles in a triangle?
8. The Pythagorean theorem relates the lengths of sides for certain triangles.

Which triangles? What is the relationship?

9. How are similar triangles defined? What is the length relationship between similar triangles?

10. What is the formula for the volume of a cube? A sphere? A cylinder?

11. What is magnification? What is the change in length, area, and volume when magnified?

PROBLEMS
Problems paralleling chapter examples

1. **(4-1)** Express 47°15′ in decimal degrees.

2. **(4-2)** Express 0.75 degrees in terms of minutes.

3. **(4-3)** An x-ray beam is directed into the angle between wall and floor. The angle between beam and floor is 30 degrees. What is the angle between the beam and wall?

4. **(4-4)** The gantry of a therapy machine is first swung 180 degrees and then 27 degrees more. What is the total angle of motion?

5. **(4-5)** An ordinary sheet of paper is about 22 × 28 cm. What is the area?

6. **(4-6)** Lead foil 1 mm thick has a mass of about 1.1 gm/cm². What is the area of foil in a 10 kg roll?

7. **(4-7)** Repeat the example, but assume the tile is 12 × 12 inches and has a contamination of 0.3 μCi while the floor size remains 10 × 12 feet.

8. **(4-8)** A ring 7 cm in diameter is made of three strands of lead wire. How many centimeters of wire did this require?

9. **(4-9)** A thin-walled cylinder of lead is 4 cm in radius and 10 cm high. If the cylinder is slit down the side and flattened out, what are the dimensions of the resulting rectangle?

10. **(4-10)** What is the area of a 6-inch image intensifier tube?

11. **(4-11)** What is the radius of the circle having the same area as a triangle with 10 cm base and 12 cm height?

12. **(4-13)** A right triangle has one angle equal to 30 degrees. What is the size of the third angle?

13. **(4-15)** The base of a certain right triangle is 12 cm and the height is 5 cm. What is the length of the hypotenuse?

14. **(4-16)** A cassette is 8 × 10 inches. What is the diagonal of this cassette? Note that this is the greatest length that can be recorded with the cassette.

15. **(4-19)** In a 30-60-90 triangle the longest side is 10 cm. How long is the shortest side?

16. **(4-22)** A pinhole camera is set up with the pinhole 20 cm from the film. If the film is exposed through the pinhole with the focal spot at 100 cm from the film, what would be the image size of a focal spot 2 × 3 mm?

17. **(4-23)** On many overhead shots, the focal-film distance is 40 inches (100 cm) and the minimum distance between the patient and the film is 4 inches (10 cm). What is the minimum magnification for any object in or on the patient?

18. **(4-24)** What is the volume (in liters) of a box 25 × 40 × 25 cm?

19. **(4-28)** What mass of water (in kilograms) would fill the box in the preceding problem?

20. **(4-37)** A solid spherical shield for the teletherapy source is 15 cm in radius. What is the volume of the material needed to form the shield?

21. **(4-41)** If the shaped block shown in Fig. 4-36 had a thickness of 12 cm on the base shown, what would have been the volume of the block?

22. **(4-42)** For an x-ray system in which the focal spot is 40 inches from the film and the table top is 4 inches from the film, what size at table top should the maximum field have when a 14 × 17 inch cassette is used?

23. **(4-45)** The maximum current for a diagnostic x-ray tube is roughly proportional to the area of the focal spot. If both the length and width of a focal spot are doubled, what factor can the current be increased by?

24. **(4-50)** At a certain distance from an x-ray tube the flux is found to be 10³ photons/cm²-sec. What is the fluence for an exposure lasting 2½ minutes?

25. **(4-54)** What is the exposure rate at 10 cm from a radium source filtered by 0.5 mm platinum that contains 10 mCi? NOTE: 1 mCi of radium is equal to 1 mg.

26. **(4-56)** A 4 cm sodium iodide (NaI) crystal is located 51 cm from a small radioactive source. What is the angle subtended by the crystal at the source?

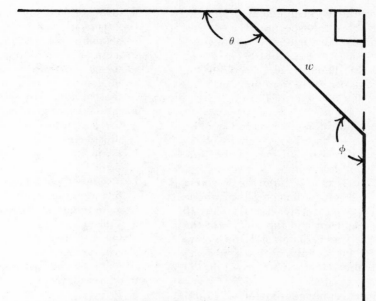

Fig. 4-45. A small wall *(w)* placed in the angle of two perpendicular walls.

27. **(4-58)** What is the solid angle subtended by the crystal, assumed to be square, at the source for the preceding problem?
28. **(4-59)** What fraction of the photons emitted in the preceding examples will impinge on the NaI crystal?

Problems related to this chapter

29. What is the smallest positive angle equal to $-30°$?
30. Express the angle $37.6°$ in degrees and minutes to the nearest minute.
31. A short diagonal wall is in the angle between two other main walls (see Fig. 4-45). If these main walls touched, they would meet in a right angle as shown in the sketch. What is the sum of the angles ϕ and θ?
32. What is the length of a diagonal (a line from one corner to the opposite corner) of a rectangle "*w*" wide and "*l*" long?
33. An ordinary piece of paper measures about 22×28 cm. If ten sheets have a mass of 42 g, what is the surface density (grams per square centimeter) of one sheet?
34. Approximately how many times can a thin wire 10 m long be wound around a pipe 5 cm in diameter?
35. A gamma camera utilizes 17 3-inch diameter photomultiplier (PM) tubes

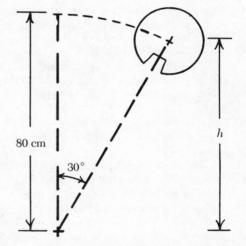

Fig. 4-46. An isocentric teletherapy machine tilted 30 degrees to the right. The height *(h)* of the source can be derived from the source axis distance (SAD) and the angle of rotation.

packed together as tightly as possible. The PM tubes just cover one side of a disc-shaped NaI crystal. What is the radius of the NaI crystal to the nearest inch?
36. In an 80 cm isocentric therapy machine the radioactive source is 80 cm from the axis of rotation of the gantry. If the gantry is rotated 30 degrees (see Fig. 4-46),

what is the vertical height (h) of the source above the isocenter?

37. An x-ray film of a patient is made with a source-image distance of 100 cm. A ring 10 cm in diameter is placed on the patient's skin 30 cm from the film. What will be the diameter of the ring on the film?

38. The magnification of a certain x-ray film is known to be 1.25. A certain object covers an area of 2.6 cm² of the film. What is the true area?

39. In a gamma camera system the detecting crystal is 30 cm in diameter, the cathode ray tube display of the crystal area is 10 cm in diameter, and the picture of the display is 4 cm in diameter. If the picture has a count density of 100 spots/cm², what is the actual count density in the detecting crystal?

40. How many cubic centimeters of liquid are needed to fill a "flood" phantom in the shape of a disc 45 cm in diameter and 0.5 cm thick?

41. ^{60}Co emits two photons per decay. What is the photon flux (in photons per square centimeter) at a distance 1 cm from a point source of 1 mCi of ^{60}Co? There are 3.7×10^7 decays per second in 1 mCi.

42. What is the solid angle subtended by the sky to an observer on a flat, treeless prairie?

43. What is the solid angle subtended by a page 15 × 18 cm held 30 cm from the eye?

44. A Geiger counter held 1 m from a source records 325 counts/min. If held 30 cm away, what would the count rate be?

45. Calculate the areas and indicate the correct units (for example, a 3 × 4 cm rectangle has an area of 12 cm²) for the following:

a. a square 6 cm on a side
b. a rectangle 4 × 10 m
c. a square with a 5 cm diagonal
d. a circle 10 feet in radius
e. the curved surface of a cylinder 10 cm long and 6 cm in diameter
f. the curved surface of a hemisphere, radius 5 cm
g. the flat surface of a hemisphere, radius 5 cm
h. a triangle of base 5 cm and height 7 cm
i. a square 6 cm on a side with a circle 6 cm in diameter removed
j. an equilateral triangle with 10 cm sides

46. Using a protractor measure the angles shown in Fig. 4-47.

47. Change the following angles in radians to degrees (for instance, $\pi/2 = 90°$):

a. π c. $\pi/12$
b. $2\pi/3$ d. $3\pi/4$

48. Evaluate the angles indicated ($\alpha, \beta, \gamma, \delta$) in Fig. 4-48. (NOTE: the figure is not to scale.)

49. Evaluate the volume for the situations indicated. As an example, the volume of a hemisphere with a 10 cm radius is 2,094 cm³:

a. a lead brick 2 × 4 × 8 inches
b. a pyramid 1 m high on a square base 1 × 1 m
c. a sphere 1 cm in diameter
d. a cylinder of $l = d = 1$ m

50. A certain object is to weigh 1 kg. Find the volume (in cubic centimeters and liters) if it is made out of each of the following (for example, air $V = 7.7 \times 10^5$ cm³ $= 7.7 \times 10^2$ liters):

a. lead   b. water
          c. aluminum

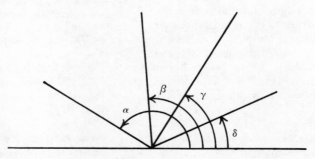

Fig. 4-47. Angles.

Objective questions

51. A right angle is
    a. 30°
    b. 45°
    c. 60°
    d. 90°
    e. 180°

52. An angle of $\pi/3$ radian measure is
    a. 30°
    b. 45°
    c. 60°
    d. 90°
    e. 180°

53. The triangle having sides 3 cm, 4 cm, and 5 cm is a right triangle. The area of the triangle is
    a. 3.5 cm²
    b. 6 cm²
    c. 7 cm²
    d. 7.5 cm²
    e. 10 cm²

54. A circle is 10 cm in diameter. The circumference is approximately
    a. 0.314 cm
    b. 3.14 cm
    c. 31.4 cm
    d. 314 cm
    e. 98.6 cm

55. A certain triangle has one right angle and one 30° angle. The other angle is
    a. 30°   d. 90°
    b. 45°   e. 180°
    c. 60°

56. In a certain right triangle the shortest side is 6 cm long. The medium length side is 8 cm long. The longest side (the hypotenuse) is
    a. 6 cm
    b. 8 cm
    c. 10 cm
    d. 12 cm
    e. 14 cm

57. Ann is 5.5 feet tall. If she stands halfway between a light bulb and a wall and if all her shadow is on the wall, how tall is her shadow?
    a. 2.75 feet
    b. 5.5 feet
    c. 8.25 feet
    d. 11 feet
    e. 22 feet

58. A certain block is 20 × 10 × 5 cm. The area of the largest side is
    a. 25 cm²
    b. 50 cm
    c. 100 cm²
    d. 200 cm²
    e. 1,000 cm²

59. Two lines cross, making an angle of 60°. They also make an angle of
    a. 30°
    b. 45°
    c. 90°
    d. 120°
    e. 170°

60. A pair of similar triangles always have
    a. right angles
    b. angles of equal magnitude

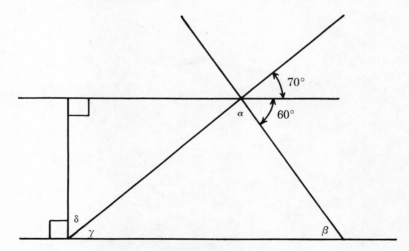

Fig. 4-48. Straight lines and angles. Geometric theorems can often be used to evaluate angles when sufficient geometric data are supplied. Figure is not to scale.

    c. angles that add to 120°
    d. obtuse angles
    e. sides of equal length

61. At 40 cm from the focal spot of an x-ray tube, a field measures 10 × 12 cm. At 60 cm this field would measure:
    a. 5 × 6 cm
    b. 6.7 × 8 cm
    c. 10 × 12 cm
    d. 12 × 16 cm
    e. 15 × 18 cm

62. One side of a right triangle has length 1 and the hypotenuse is 2. The length of the other side is
    a. $x = 1$
    b. $x = \sqrt{2}$
    c. $x = \sqrt{3}$
    d. $x = 2$
    e. $x = 3$

63. The area of a circle 2 cm in diameter is approximately
    a. 3.14 cm²
    b. 4 cm²
    c. 6.28 cm²
    d. 8 cm²
    e. 12.56 cm²

64. An adult 66 inches tall will weigh _____ times a child 33 inches tall.
    a. 1
    b. 2
    c. 3
    d. 4
    e. 8

CHAPTER 5

Trigonometry

Trigonometry—literally "triangle measurement"— is the study of the properties of triangles. An extension of plane geometry (Chapter 4), it is often applied to a variety of situations involving angles. It is also used in many scientific and engineering problems, such as rotations and wave motion, whose relationship to angles and plane geometry is not so obvious.

TRIGONOMETRIC RATIOS

Trigonometric ratios or *functions* are the relations between any two sides of a right triangle, involving an acute angle of a given size.

FUNCTIONS. Fig. 5-1 shows two right triangles that have a common acute angle α. The other acute angle in both triangles must be $90° - \alpha$, since all the angles in a triangle add up to 180 degrees. Triangles that have equal corresponding angles—like these two—are called similar, and any ratio between the sides in one such triangle is equal to the corresponding ratio in the other. For example, the ratio x/r is equal to X/R, and for all right triangles with an angle equal to α, the corresponding ratio equals the ratio for either of the triangles shown in Fig. 5-1. Hence in a right triangle with a specified acute angle, the ratios between the sides are fixed.

With respect to a given acute angle in a right triangle (such as α in Fig. 5-1), the sides are called *opposite* (y) and *adjacent* (x). The side opposite the right angle is the hypotenuse (r). Six ratios can be conceived of for a triangle: y/r, x/r, y/x, r/x, r/y, and x/y. Each of these ratios corresponds to a trigonometric function. Three of them are the inverse of the other three. The three most commonly used are called *sine, cosine,* and *tangent.* They are defined as follows:

$$\text{Sine of } \alpha = \frac{\text{Opposite}}{\text{Hypotenuse}} = \boxed{\sin \alpha = y/r} \qquad \textbf{Formula 5-1}$$

$$\text{Cosine of } \alpha = \frac{\text{Adjacent}}{\text{Hypotenuse}} = \boxed{\cos \alpha = x/r} \qquad \textbf{Formula 5-2}$$

$$\text{Tangent of } \alpha = \frac{\text{Opposite}}{\text{Adjacent}} = \boxed{\tan \alpha = y/x} \qquad \textbf{Formula 5-3}$$

These definitions should be memorized. The other three are usually expressed in terms of the first three ratios as follows:

$$\text{Cosecant of } \alpha = \csc \alpha = \frac{1}{\sin \alpha}$$

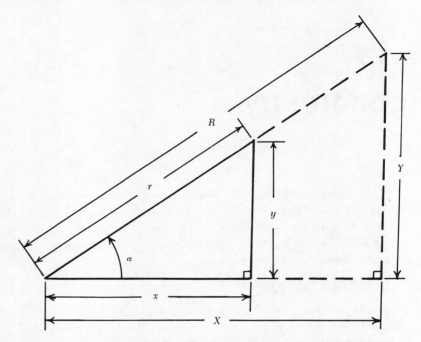

Fig. 5-1. Two right triangles, sharing the same acute angle α. These triangles must be "similar"; the ratios in one triangle, such as x/y, must equal the corresponding ratio $s(x/y)$ in the other, X/Y.

$$\text{Secant of } \alpha = \sec \alpha = \frac{1}{\cos \alpha}$$

$$\text{Cotangent of } \alpha = \cot \alpha = \frac{1}{\tan \alpha}$$

The practical application of trigonometric ratios will be discussed later in this chapter. Only one example shall be given here.

Example 5-1. Fig. 4-26 in Chapter 4 showed that in a 45-45-90 triangle the ratio of the sides is $1:1:\sqrt{2}$. What are the trigonometric functions sin 45°, cos 45°, and tan 45°? The sine is equal to the opposite divided by the hypotenuse, or $\sin 45° = \frac{1}{\sqrt{2}}$. The cosine is equal to the adjacent divided by the hypotenuse, or $\cos 45° = \frac{1}{\sqrt{2}}$. The tangent is equal the opposite divided by the adjacent, or $\tan 45° = 1$.

NEGATIVE AND OBTUSE ANGLES. Fig. 5-2 shows a negative acute angle (θ) in a right triangle placed with side x along the horizontal axis in the positive direction (to the right of the origin) and with side y parallel to the vertical axis in the negative direction (downward from the horizontal axis) (Chapter 6). The hypotenuse ($r = \sqrt{x^2 + y^2}$) is positive in all triangles. Because y is negative and x and r are positive, the sine and tangent functions will be negative whereas the cosine function will remain positive. The absolute value of all

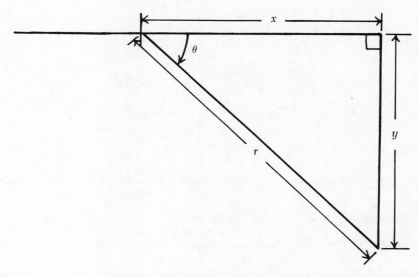

Fig. 5-2. A right triangle containing the negative acute angle θ. The length y is considered negative, whereas x and r are positive.

three ratios is the same as the value for the positive angles of the same magnitude. Expressed as formulas, this is as follows:

$$\sin(-\theta) = -\sin \theta \qquad \text{Formula 5-4}$$

$$\cos(-\theta) = \cos \theta \qquad \text{Formula 5-5}$$

$$\tan(-\theta) = -\tan \theta \qquad \text{Formula 5-6}$$

Example 5-2. In example 5-1 we determined the trigonometric functions for $\alpha = +45°$. What are these functions for -45 degrees? The relationships given show that $\sin(-45°) = -\sin 45° = \dfrac{-1}{\sqrt{2}}$; $\cos(-45°) = \cos 45° = \dfrac{1}{\sqrt{2}}$; $\tan(-45°) = -\tan 45° = -1$.

Obtuse angles cannot exist within a right triangle.

By definition, the absolute value of the trigonometric ratios for an obtuse angle is the same as that for its supplementary angle (two angles are supplementary when their sum is 180 degrees). In other words, the ratios of an angle and the ratios of its supplement have the same magnitude and may differ only by their sign. As shown in Fig. 5-3, for any angle θ between 90 and 180 degrees, the value of x is negative and that of y is positive. Thus the sine of θ is positive and equal to the sine of $\phi = 180* - \theta$, the supplement of θ; the

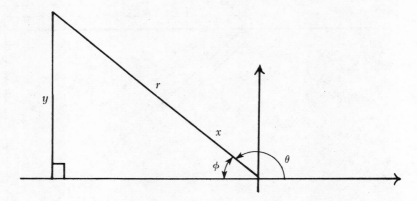

Fig. 5-3. The trigonometric ratios for the obtuse angle θ. Because θ cannot be an internal angle of a right triangle, it is considered an *external* angle. The ratios for θ and for ϕ are defined as the same; note, however, that ϕ is not in standard position and that x is negative.

cosine of θ is negative and the tangent of θ is also negative. Expressed as formulas we have:

$$\sin(\theta) = \sin(180° - \theta) \qquad\qquad \text{Formula 5-7}$$

$$\cos(\theta) = -\cos(180° - \theta) \qquad\qquad \text{Formula 5-8}$$

$$\tan(\theta) = -\tan(180° - \theta) \qquad\qquad \text{Formula 5-9}$$

Example 5-3. Use the values obtained in Example 5-1 to find the trigonometric functions for 135 degrees, the supplement of 45 degrees. The relationships above show that $\sin 135° = \sin 45° = \dfrac{1}{\sqrt{2}}$; $\cos 135° = -\cos 45° = -\dfrac{1}{\sqrt{2}}$, and $\tan 135° = -\tan 45° = -1$.

IDENTITIES. Trigonometric identities are relationships between trigonometric functions that are *true for any angle*. The relationships introduced in the previous section (formulas 5-4 through 5-9) are examples of trigonometric identities.

They have various uses, from the simplification of formulas to the practical utilization of tabulated trigonometric data ("trig tables"). The latter application has been seen in examples 5-2 and 5-3. Generally, trigonometric functions are only tabulated for angles between 0 and 90 degrees; for other angles the functions must be found by the formulas listed in the preceding section of this chapter.

Example 5-4. Find the value of cos 153° in terms of the functions of an angle between 0 and 90 degrees. Here the obtuse angle formula (formula 5-8) can be used. Cos 153° = $-\cos(180° - 153°)$ = $-\cos 27°$.

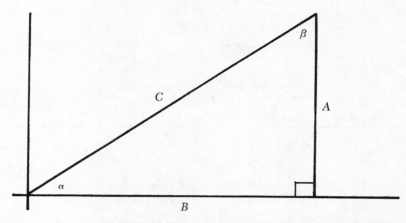

Fig. 5-4. Complementary angles. The angles α and β add to 90 degrees and are thus *complementary*. The cosine of α is *B/C;* this is equal to the sine of β.

Example 5-5. Express sin 220° in terms of the functions of an angle between 0 and 90 degrees. First we can use the obtuse angle formula (formula 5-7): sin 220° = sin(180° − 220°) = sin(−40°); then the negative angle formula (formula 5-4) gives sin(−40°) = −sin 40°. Thus sin 220° = −sin 40°.

Another important group of identities involves *complementary* angles. As explained in Chapter 4, two angles are complementary when their sum is 90 degrees. In a right triangle the acute angles are always complementary and the *opposite* (side) of one acute angle is the *adjacent* of the other. Hence the sine of one angle is equal to the cosine of the other. This can be formulated as follows:

$$\sin \theta = \cos(90° − \theta)$$ **Formula 5-10**

$$\cos \theta = \sin(90° − \theta)$$ **Formula 5-11**

The tangent of one of the acute angles is the inverse of the tangent of the complementary angle or:

$$\tan(\theta) = \frac{1}{\tan(90° − \theta)} = \cot(90° − \theta)$$ **Formula 5-12**

These relationships between complementary angles can be used to further reduce the size of trigonometric tables. This is commonly done in one of two ways. In one, the sine, cosine, and tangent can be given for angles from 0 to 45 degrees; the complementary angle formulas are used to evaluate the functions for the angles between 45 and 90 degrees. In the other, only the sine and tangent are given for angles from 0 to 90 degrees; the cosine is found by the complementary angle formulas.

Table 3

Values of some trigonometric functions

θ (degrees)	Sin θ	Cos θ	Tan θ	Cot θ
0	0	1	0	∞
1	0.0175	0.9998	0.0175	57.29
2	0.0349	0.9994	0.0349	28.64
3	0.0523	0.9986	0.0524	19.08
4	0.0698	0.9976	0.0699	14.30
5	0.0872	0.9962	0.0875	11.43
6	0.1045	0.9945	0.1051	9.514
7	0.1219	0.9925	0.1228	8.144
8	0.1392	0.9903	0.1405	7.115
9	0.1564	0.9877	0.1584	6.314
10	0.1736	0.9848	0.1763	5.671
11	0.1908	0.9816	0.1944	5.145
12	0.2079	0.9781	0.2126	4.705
13	0.2250	0.9744	0.2309	4.331
14	0.2419	0.9703	0.2493	4.011
15	0.2588	0.9659	0.2679	3.732
16	0.2756	0.9613	0.2867	3.487
17	0.2924	0.9563	0.3057	3.271
18	0.3090	0.9511	0.3249	3.078
19	0.3256	0.9455	0.3443	2.904
20	0.3420	0.9397	0.3640	2.747
21	0.3584	0.9336	0.3839	2.605
22	0.3746	0.9272	0.4040	2.475
23	0.3907	0.9205	0.4245	2.356
24	0.4067	0.9135	0.4452	2.246
25	0.4226	0.9063	0.4663	2.145
26	0.4384	0.8988	0.4877	2.050
27	0.4540	0.8910	0.5095	1.963
28	0.4695	0.8829	0.5317	1.881
29	0.4848	0.8746	0.5543	1.804
30	0.5000	0.8660	0.5774	1.732
31	0.5150	0.8572	0.6009	1.664
32	0.5299	0.8480	0.6249	1.600
33	0.5446	0.8387	0.6494	1.540
34	0.5592	0.8290	0.6745	1.483
35	0.5736	0.8192	0.7002	1.428
36	0.5878	0.8090	0.7265	1.376
37	0.6018	0.7986	0.7536	1.327
38	0.6157	0.7880	0.7813	1.280
39	0.6293	0.7771	0.8098	1.235
40	0.6428	0.7660	0.8391	1.192
41	0.6561	0.7547	0.8693	1.150
42	0.6691	0.7431	0.9004	1.111
43	0.6820	0.7314	0.9325	1.072
44	0.6947	0.7193	0.9657	1.036
45	0.7071	0.7071	1.0000	1.000

Example 5-6. Find cos 48.6°. What functions should we look up in a table containing only the sine and tangent functions? The complementary angle formula (formula 5-11) shows that cos 48.6° = sin(90° − 48.6°) = sin 41.4°.

There are numerous other identities, including addition and subtraction of angles and half-angle and double-angle relationships, that can be found in mathematical handbooks. The techniques of their derivation are explained in standard texts.

VALUES OF TRIGONOMETRIC FUNCTIONS. In our work, we are mainly concerned with the numerical values of trigonometric functions. Although these values can be mathematically derived, we shall simply use the values shown in Table 3, except for the special angles discussed here.

Special angles. The value of the trigonometric functions for the angles 0, 30, 45, 60, and 90 degrees can be determined by using principles of geometry. Some of this was done in examples 5-1 and 5-2. In reality, no triangle can have an angle of 0 degrees. However, we can conceive of one with a very small acute angle that approaches zero (Fig. 5-5); in this case the opposite side is very small. Conceptually, it is reasonable to assume that it is of zero length; then, sin 0° = 0. Also, the adjacent side will coincide with the hypotenuse and thus cos 0° = 1.

Example 5-7. What is tan 0°? $\tan 0° = \dfrac{\text{opposite}}{\text{adjacent}} = \dfrac{y}{x} = \dfrac{y/r}{x/r} = \dfrac{\sin 0°}{\cos 0°}$

$= \dfrac{0}{1} = 0.$

In a similar way, we can construct a triangle in which the acute angle is almost 90 degrees and from this we can obtain the functions for 90 degrees. These values can also be found by using the identities presented earlier in this chapter (see discussion of trigonometric identities). Thus sin 90° = cos (90° − 90°) = cos 0° = 1; cos 90° = sin(90° − 90°) = sin 0° = 0. Tan 90° = $\dfrac{1}{\tan(90° − 90°)} = \dfrac{1}{\tan 0°} = 1/0$; this ratio is an immeasurably large amount called infinity and represented by the symbol ∞. It is important to

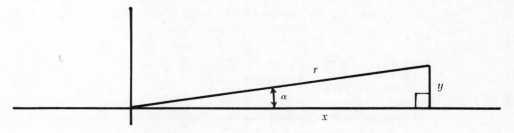

Fig. 5-5. A triangle with a very small angle. If the angle α is very small, y will be very small compared to x and r; and x and r will also be approximately equal.

become familiar with the values of the trigonometric ratios for the most frequently used angles. For convenience, some of these are tabulated here:

Angle	Sine	Cosine	Tangent
0°	0	1	0
30°	$\frac{1}{2}$	$\frac{\sqrt{3}}{2}$	$\frac{1}{\sqrt{3}}$
45°	$\frac{1}{\sqrt{2}}$	$\frac{1}{\sqrt{2}}$	1
60°	$\frac{\sqrt{3}}{2}$	$\frac{1}{2}$	$\sqrt{3}$
90°	1	0	∞

Trigonometric tables. We have seen that *exact* expressions exist for the trigonometric ratios of certain special angles. For others, *approximate* values can be developed to any practical level of accuracy desired. These can be found in trigonometric tables such as Table 3.

> **Example 5-8.** What is the value of sin 11°? In Table 3, this is read directly from the second column of row 11; the value is 0.1908.

In some cases we have to utilize one or more trigonometric identities for the solution.

> **Example 5-9.** What is the value of tan 55°? Table 3 only covers up to 45 degrees. But we can use the identity $\tan 55° = \dfrac{1}{\tan(90° - 55°)} = \dfrac{1}{\tan 35°}$; find tan 35° from the table as 0.7002, and then take the inverse. Or we can look up the cotangent, since $\dfrac{1}{\tan 35°} = \cot 35° = 1.428$.

If it is necessary to find trigonometric values for intermediate angles, we use a method called "interpolation." Here we will consider only values that are halfway between the tabulated values. In Chapter 11, we apply this method to other intermediate values. To find a value midway between two tabulated values, compute their average.

> **Example 5-10.** Using Table 3, find the value of cos 34.5°. By interpolation: $\cos 34.5° \cong \dfrac{\cos 34° + \cos 35°}{2} = \dfrac{0.8290 + 0.8192}{2} = 0.8241$.

Inverse functions. The ordinary trigonometric function expresses the value of the ratio between two sides of a right triangle, provided the value of one of the acute angles is known. For example, if a right triangle has an angle of 30 degrees, then sin 30° = $\frac{1}{2}$ tells us that one of its sides is half the length of the hypotenuse. The converse is also true: if in a right triangle one side is half the length of the hypotenuse, then one of the angles is 30 degrees. This is expressed formally by the *inverse* trigonometric function—in our example sin^{-1} $\frac{1}{2}$ = 30°—and read as "the angle whose sine is $\frac{1}{2}$ is equal to 30 degrees" or "the inverse sine of $\frac{1}{2}$ is 30 degrees."

Note that here "$^{-1}$" does not mean the negative exponent one, but rather the inverse functional operation, for example:

$$\sin^{-1}(\sin\,\theta) = \theta$$

Many practitioners prefer to use the prefix "arc" to indicate an inverse. For example, arctan x is the same as tan^{-1}x.

Some mathematical tables include inverse trigonometric functions, but usually these must be looked for in regular trigonometric tables.

> **Example 5-11.** Find sin^{-1}(0.36) to the nearest degree. For this we can simply run our finger down the column of sin θ in Table 3 until we find approximately 0.36. This is seen to be approximately at the angle 21 degrees.

PRACTICAL APPLICATIONS OF TRIGONOMETRY

In general, trigonometry is applied only in practical situations. Even a great deal of practical geometry utilizes trigonometry, particularly for unusual angles or geometric shapes. But because trigonometry is based on the right triangle, and other triangles must, for that purpose, be divided into a pair of right triangles. Of course, any plane geometric figure with straight sides can be sectioned into triangles.

SOLUTION OF RIGHT TRIANGLES. The most direct application of trigonometry is in the *solution* of right triangles. "Solution" here means information about other values such as area.

In order to "solve" a right triangle we need to know two values other than the fact that one angle is 90 degrees. We must know the length of one side and either the measurement of one angle or the length of another side. An example of a solvable right triangle is shown in Fig. 5-6. The full solution requires the determination of the angle θ and the lengths R and x. In this type of problem the angle θ is most easily found. Since θ is complementary to 35 degrees, $\theta = 90° - 35° = 55°$. The lengths are determined by the following trigonometric ratios:

$$\frac{5}{R} = \cos 35°$$
$$R = \frac{5}{\cos 35°} = \frac{5}{0.8192} = 6.1 \text{ cm}$$

$$\frac{x}{5} = \tan 35°$$
$$x = 5 \tan 35° = 5 \times 0.7002 = 3.5 \text{ cm}$$

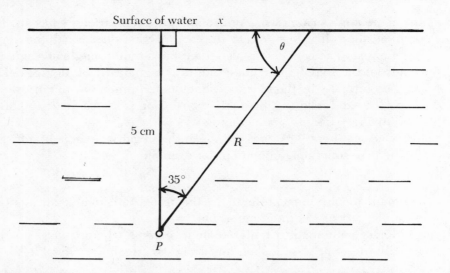

Fig. 5-6. A point *(P)* is 5 cm below the surface of a water phantom. If one of the acute angles is known (35 degrees), the distance *(R)* from the point to the surface can be found.

This completes the solution of the triangle. In most practical cases like this we do not really need the whole solution, but only one or two of the parameters.

> **Example 5-12.** A photon beam traverses a concrete wall 1 m thick at the angle shown in Fig. 5-7. Solve the triangle made by the beam, the dotted line, and the upper surface of the wall. This is a right triangle with a height of 1 m and an angle of 43 degrees opposite the height. The other angle is $90° - 43° = 47°$. The hypotenuse is $\dfrac{1}{\sin 43°} = 1.47$ and the base is $\dfrac{1}{\tan 43°} = 1.07$ m.

Right triangles with two sides of known length can be solved by straight-forward application of the trigonometric ratios.

> **Example 5-13.** Solve the right triangles formed by bisecting the triangle shown in Fig. 5-8. This leads to two right triangles, each with a base of 10 cm and a height of 100 cm. The hypotenuse is $\sqrt{10{,}100} \cong 100.5$ cm. The angle ϕ is $\tan^{-1}(^{10}/_{100}) \cong 5.7°$; the other angle is 84.3 degrees. The angular aperture γ is 2ϕ, or $11.4°$.

> **Example 5-14.** Draw a 20-degree angle without a protractor. You can do this by using the trigonometric ratios and a piece of graph paper. In a right triangle with an angle of 20 degrees, the ratio of the opposite

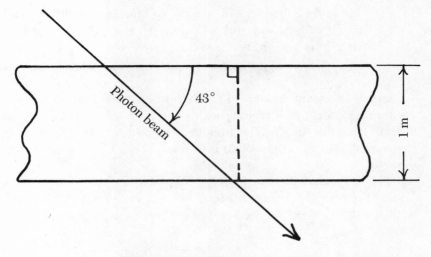

Fig. 5-7. A ray traverses a wall 1 m thick.

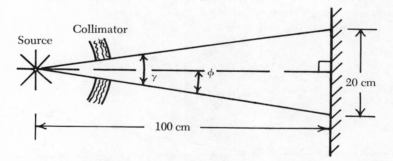

Fig. 5-8. A beam is 20 cm wide at 100 cm from a point source (focal spot or a radioactive source). What is the angular aperture (γ) of the collimators?

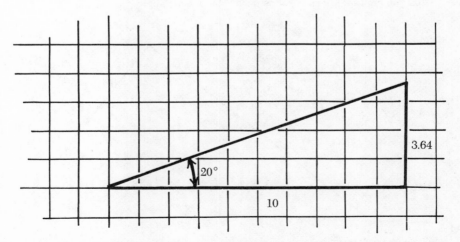

Fig. 5-9. Constructing a 20-degree angle. Any angle can be drawn using a right angle and the trigonometric ratios.

side to the adjacent side should be equal to tan 20° = 0.364. Hence a height of 3.64 cm and a base of 10 cm would be appropriate. The triangle is shown in Fig. 5-9.

Law of sines and cosines. Fig. 5-10 represents a collimated x-ray beam with an angular aperture of 12 degrees directed on a cassette whose near edge is 100 cm from the source. The cassette is tipped so that it forms an angle of 104 degrees at the near edge. What is the height (Z) of the beam projected on the cassette?

This is an example in which the "law of sines" can be used. But let us first look at the triangle shown in Fig. 5-11 with angles *a*, *b*, and *c*, and sides *A*, *B*, and *C*. For this triangle the law of sines reads as follows:

$$\frac{A}{\sin a} = \frac{B}{\sin b} = \frac{C}{\sin c}$$

Formula 5-13

With this relationship the triangle in Fig. 5-10 is readily solved. The angle opposite the 100 cm side is 180° − 12° − 104° = 64°. The law of sines in this case shows that:

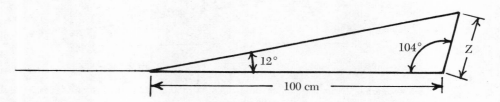

Fig. 5-10. The projection of a 12-degree beam on an angled cassette. Because this is not a right triangle, the trigonometric ratios cannot be directly applied.

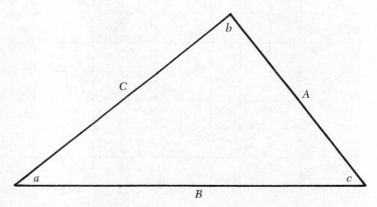

Fig. 5-11. A triangle labeled for illustration of the law of sines and the law of cosines. In this triangle side *A* is opposite angle *a*, side *B* is opposite angle *b*, and side *C* is opposite angle *c*.

$$\frac{Z}{\sin 12°} = \frac{100}{\sin 64°}$$

$$Z = 100 \, \frac{\sin 12°}{\sin 64°}$$

$$Z = 100 \times \frac{0.2079}{0.8988} = 23.1 \text{ cm}$$

Similarly, the longest side is:

$$100 \times \frac{\sin 104°}{\sin 64°} = 100 \times \frac{0.9703}{0.8988} = 108.0 \text{ cm}$$

Example 5-15. Find the path length of the x-ray shown in Fig. 5-12. In the triangle defined by the electron path, the x-ray, and the anode surface the angles are 76, 100, and 4 degrees. The 1 mm side is opposite the 4-degree angle and the side whose length we want to find is opposite the 76-degree angle. Therefore the length of this side is equal to

$$1 \times \frac{\sin 76°}{\sin 4°} = \frac{0.9703}{0.0698} = 13.9 \text{ mm.}$$

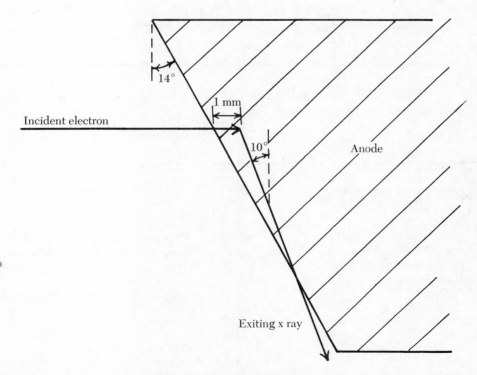

Fig. 5-12. An x ray produced by an incident electron hitting an anode at a depth of 1 mm. How far will the x ray travel in the anode? X rays are produced at many depths and travel in many different directions. The angles in this figure have been exaggerated.

The law of sines is particularly useful when an angle and an opposite side are known in addition to another angle or another side. Another formula, the *law of cosines*, is useful when three sides of a triangle or two sides and the contained angle are known. This formula (angles and sides labeled as in Fig. 5-11) is:

$$2AB \cos c = A^2 + B^2 - C^2 \qquad\qquad \text{Formula 5-14}$$

> **Example 5-16.** Use formula 5-14 to show that in an equilateral triangle all angles are 60 degrees. Call the length of each side S. Then, formula 5-14 becomes $2S^2 \cos c = S^2 + S^2 - S^2 = S^2$; then $\cos c = \dfrac{S^2}{2S^2} = \dfrac{1}{2}$; and $c = 60$ degrees.

Here we use the cosine law to find an angle when all the sides of a triangle are known. The next example shows the situation where we know two sides and the contained angle.

> **Example 5-17.** Solve formula 5-14 for the side C. The formula can be rewritten as $C^2 = A^2 + B^2 - 2AB \cos c$. The square root of both sides is taken, with the positive root retained as $C = \sqrt{A^2 + B^2 - 2AB \cos c}$.

The law of sines and the law of cosines apply to all triangles, including those with right and obtuse angles.

CHAPTER REVIEW

1. What are the definitions of sine, cosine, and tangent in terms of adjacent, opposite, and hypotenuse?
2. How are the ratios of a negative angle defined?
3. How are the ratios defined for obtuse angles?
4. What is a trigonometric identity?
5. What are *complementary* and *supplementary* angles?
6. What is interpolation?
7. What is an inverse trigonometric function?

8. What is the *solution* of a triangle?
9. What type of triangle can be solved by direct application of the trigonometric ratio definitions?
10. What are the two formulas called that are used for solving general triangles?

PROBLEMS
Problems paralleling chapter examples

1. (5-1) In Chapter 4 it was shown that a 30-60-90 triangle had sides with the ratio $2:\sqrt{3}:1$. The shortest side is opposite the

30 degree angle. What are the trigonometric functions for 30 degrees?

2. (5-2) What are the trigonometric functions for −30 degrees?

3. (5-3) Use the values obtained in problem 1 to express the functions of 150 degrees.

4. (5-4) Express sin 127° in terms of the functions of an angle between 0 and 90 degrees.

5. (5-5) Express cos 265° in terms of the functions of an angle between 0 and 90 degrees.

6. (5-8) What is tan 25°?

7. (5-9) What is sin 67°?

8. (5-10) Find the value of tan 15.5° by interpolation.

9. (5-11) Find $\cos^{-1} 0.92$.

10. (5-12) Solve the triangle in Fig. 5-7 assuming the angle shown is 48 degrees instead of 43 degrees.

11. (5-13) A therapy beam is 15 cm wide on the patient's skin 80 cm from the source. What is the angular aperture of the collimator?

12. (5-14) We wish to draw a 37 degree angle. If the angle is to be in standard position and the base is 10.0 cm, what height must it have?

13. (5-15) Repeat example 5-15 with the 10-degree angle changed to 5 degrees, the angulation remaining 14 degrees, and the depth 1 mm.

14. (5-16) Use formula 5-14 to show that the triangle whose sides are in the ratio of 5:12:13 is a right triangle.

Problems related to this chapter

15. A ramp is made with a "1 in 10" incline (one vertical unit for ten horizontal units). What is the angle of the ramp to the horizontal?

16. Obtain numerical values for:
    a. sin 34°
    b. cos(−16°)
    c. tan 127°
    d. sin 541°

17. Solve the triangle whose sides are 3, 4, and 5 cm long.

18. A triangle has sides 7, 8, and 9 cm long. Find the area of the triangle and the size of the smallest angle.

19. In a focused grid the grid lines run parallel to the x-rays. Find the angle of incli-

nation in relation to a line parallel to the central ray for a line 10 cm from the center of a focused grid intended for use at 100 cm.

20. A right triangle has a hypotenuse 15 cm long and one angle of 48 degrees. Solve the triangle.

21. In the usual geometry of an x-ray tube in which the useful x-ray beam is at right angles to the incident electrons, the apparent focal spot width is the true width multiplied by sin θ, where θ is the angle between the anode and the useful beam. What is the true width of a 0.8 mm (apparent) focal spot angulated at 12 degrees.

22. If sin θ = 0.35, what is cos θ?

23. In a six-pulse, three-phase circuit, the minimum voltage V_{min} is related to the peak voltage V_p as follows:

$$\frac{V_{min}}{V_p} = \frac{\sin 90° + \sin 30°}{2 \sin 60°}$$

Express V_{min} as a percent of V_p.

24. The change in wavelength ($\Delta\lambda$) for a photon scattered by the Compton process is:

$$\Delta\lambda = 0.0243(1 - \cos \theta)$$

where θ is the scattering angle and the wavelength is in angstroms (10^{-10} m). Find the change in wavelength for 0, 90, and 180 degree scattering angles.

25. A thin strip of lead 1 cm wide is tilted so that it makes an angle of 38 degrees with the incident x-ray beam. How wide is the shadow of the strip on an x-ray film placed immediately behind the strip?

26. A parallelogram has two sides of 10 cm and two of 15 cm. If one diagonal is 20 cm long, what is the length of the other diagonal?

Objective questions

27. The cos −20° is equal to:
    a. sin −20°
    b. cos 20°
    c. $\cos^{-1} 20°$
    d. sin 20°
    e. sin −70°

28. "The angle whose sine is 0.65" can also be written as:
    a. $\sin^{-1} 0.65$
    b. inversine 0.65

c. $\dfrac{1}{\sin 0.65}$

d. cosine 0.65

e. arccos 0.65

29. Sin 20 degrees is equal to:
    a. $-\cos 20°$
    b. $\sin 70°$
    c. $-\sin 70°$
    d. $\sin -20°$
    e. $\cos 70°$

30. Cos 0° is equal to:
    a. 0
    b. ½
    c. $1/\sqrt{2}$
    d. $\dfrac{\sqrt{3}}{2}$
    e. 1

31. The value of $\cos^{-1}(\cos \theta)$ is equal to:
    a. θ
    b. $\sin \theta$
    c. $\cos \theta$
    d. 1
    e. an undefined quantity

32. In a right triangle of hypotenuse (R) containing the acute angle $\theta > 45°$, the shortest side is:
    a. $R \sin \theta$
    b. $R \cos \theta$
    c. $R \tan \theta$
    d. $\dfrac{R}{\sin \theta}$
    e. $\dfrac{R}{\cos \theta}$

33. A triangle with the length of the three sides given is to be solved. The most useful relationship for the first step of the solution is the use of the:
    a. law of sines
    b. law of cosines
    c. Pythagorean theorem
    d. trigonometric ratios
    e. inverse trigonometric functions

34. A right triangle has a hypotenuse of 10 cm and an angle of 35 degrees; ($\sin 35° = 0.57$, $\cos 35° = 0.82$, $\tan 35° = 0.70$). The area of this triangle is about:
    a. 20 cm²
    b. 23 cm²
    c. 29 cm²
    d. 35 cm²
    e. 72 cm²

35. A beam of radiation strikes a wall 0.5 m thick at an angle of 30 degrees. The path of the beam in the wall is about:
    a. 0.3 m
    b. 0.7 m
    c. 0.9 m
    d. 1.0 m
    e. 1.4 m

CHAPTER 6

Graphic display

When a table contains more than about five entries, it becomes difficult to interpret the tabulated data. Similarly, when an algebraic function contains several terms, it is difficult to interpret even some of the gross features of the relationship. One approach to the interpretation of algebraic functions is offered by the calculus (Chapter 10); another is by using a *graph*, in which numerical values are represented as positions in a plane. This reduces a typical functional relationship to a curved or straight line. Instead of the generally unappealing formulas of algebra, we now have a picture. In general, this is easier to understand than the tabular or algebraic forms.

Once a relationship is represented as a picture, the language of geometry can be utilized. The reverse can also be done, that is, geometric problems can be solved through algebra. These processes are known as *analytic geometry*.

Graphs play an important role in the evaluation of experimental investigations. Experimental data are usually recorded in tabular form. These data are often thought to represent a more or less smooth functional relationship, with fluctuations and measurement uncertainties superimposed. In fitting a line to these experimental empirical data, we try to obtain a picture of the underlying relationship.

COORDINATE SYSTEMS

A graph is a two-dimensional representation of certain quantities; lengths and angles are its major means of expression. A *coordinate system* permits us to identify any position in two-dimensional space in terms of the values of two parameters. There are many such systems.

If a position is determined completely by a single coordinate, the situation is called *one-dimensional*. For example, the position of a bead on a wire loop is completely determined by the angle formed at the center of the loop by the horizontal line and the bead's position. This is shown in Fig. 6-1. If two coordinates are required to specify a position, the system is called *two-dimensional*. *Three-dimensional systems* are also possible.

CARTESIAN SYSTEM. The *Cartesian system*, named for the mathematician René Descartes, uses lengths measured at right angles to define positions. It is shown in Fig. 6-2; the distances are measured in a horizontal and vertical direction. The horizontal distance from the y-axis to a point such as P or Q in the figure is known as the *abscissa* of the point or the x *coordinate* of the point. The vertical distance, measured from the x-axis to the point, is known as the

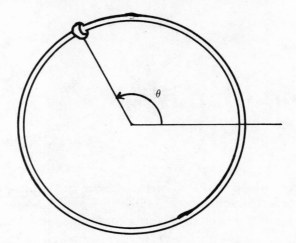

Fig. 6-1. A one-dimensional system. The bead's position on the wire ring is completely determined by the single angle θ.

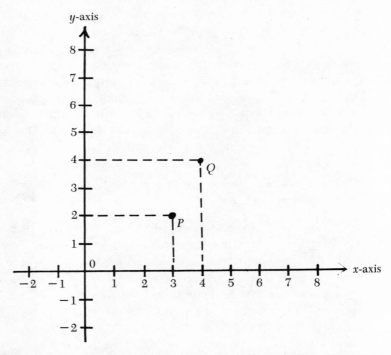

Fig. 6-2. The Cartesian coordinate system. In this system a point such as P or Q is represented by a horizontal distance, the x distance, and by a vertical distance, the y distance.

ordinate or y *coordinate* of the point. In the figure, point P has the values $x = 3$ and $y = 2$.

Example 6-1. What are the coordinates of point Q in Fig. 6-2? It can be seen that the value of x is 4 and that y is also 4.

The horizontal line having the value $y = 0$ is known as the *x-axis*. The vertical line through $x = 0$, is called the *y-axis*. The axes cross at the point $x = 0$, $y = 0$; this point is called the *origin*, often represented by a capital O.

The Cartesian coordinates give us a way to position points that are defined by a pair of values. One can also do geometric *calculations* on the points and figures defined by the points. For example, in Fig. 6-2 we can find the distance from P to Q or the angle between the x-axis and the straight line from the origin to Q.

Suppose we want to find the distance from the origin to the point P_1 of Fig. 6-3 located at $x = x_1$ and $y = y_1$: The vertical line from P_1 to the x-axis and the line from the origin to P_1 defines a right triangle with a base of length x_1 and height y_1. The distance from the origin to P_1 is the hypotenuse of this triangle. The Pythagorean theorem (formula 4-8) relates these three lengths. For this point, $r_1 = \sqrt{x_1{}^2 + y_1{}^2}$. In general, for a point at position x and y the distance(r) from the origin is as follows:

$$r = \sqrt{x^2 + y^2}$$

Formula 6-1

Example 6-2. What is the distance from the origin to point P of Fig. 6-2? Because $x = 3$ and $y = 2$, $r = \sqrt{3^2 + 2^2} = \sqrt{13} \cong 3.6$.

What about the distance between two points not including the origin? Consider r_{21} the distance between point P_1 and P_2 of Fig. 6-3. A right triangle

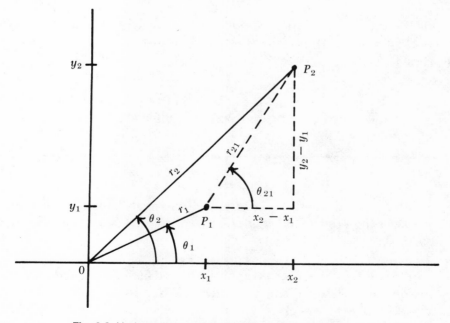

Fig. 6-3. Various distances and angles in a Cartesian system.

is defined by the vertical line from P_2, the horizontal line from P_1 and the line from P_1 to P_2. Since the base of this triangle is $x_2 - x_1$ and the height is $y_2 - y_1$, the Pythagorean theorem (formula 4-8) can be applied again with the following result:

$$r_{21} = \sqrt{(x_2 - x_1)^2 + (y_2 - y_1)^2} \qquad \text{Formula 6-2}$$

Example 6-3. What is the distance between points P $(x = 3, y = 2)$ and Q $(x = 4, y = 4)$ in Fig. 6-2? We put these values into formula 6-2 to obtain:

$$r_{PQ} = \sqrt{(4 - 3)^2 + (4 - 2)^2} = \sqrt{1^2 + 2^2} = \sqrt{1 + 4} = \sqrt{5} \cong 2.2$$

Angles can also be found fairly easily in this coordinate system. First, consider the angle θ_1, between the x-axis and the line from the origin to P_1 in Fig. 6-3. This angle is one corner of the right triangle with base x_1, height y_1, and hypotenuse r_1. Thus the definitions of the trigonometric ratios for this right triangle are:

$$\sin \theta_1 = \frac{y_1}{r_1} = \frac{y_1}{\sqrt{x_1^2 + y_1^2}}$$

$$\cos \theta_1 = \frac{x_1}{r_1} = \frac{x_1}{\sqrt{x_1^2 + y_1^2}}$$

$$\tan \theta_1 = \frac{y_1}{x_1} \qquad \text{Formula 6-3}$$

Of the three possible forms, the version involving the tangent is the most easily used. This is sometimes written in terms of the inverse function as $\theta_1 = \tan^{-1}\left(\frac{y_1}{x_1}\right)$.

Example 6-4. What is the angle between the x-axis and the line from the origin to P in Fig. 6-2? The angle θ obeys the formula $\tan \theta = \frac{2}{3}$, or $\theta \cong 33.7$ degrees.

Similar arguments can be used to find the angle between lines that do not intersect the origin. For example, it can be seen in Fig. 6-3 that $\theta_{21} = \tan^{-1}\frac{(y_2 - y_1)}{(x_2 - x_1)}$.

Everything done so far has been illustrated in the *first quadrant* of the space divided into four quadrants by the x and y axes, that is, with positive values of x and y only. However, all the formulas hold also for the other quadrants, provided all quantities are entered with their appropriate algebraic sign.

Example 6-5. Find the distance from the point $x_1 = -2$, $y_1 = -3$ and the point $x_2 = -1$, $y_2 = +1$. These values are inserted into formula 6-2 to obtain

$$r = \sqrt{[-1 + 2]^2 + [1 + 3]^2} = \sqrt{1^2 + 4^2} = \sqrt{17} \cong 4.1$$

The most important geometric quantities, distances and angles, can be found in a fairly straightforward manner using Cartesian coordinates. For this reason Cartesian coordinates are by far the most popular and most useful of the coordinate systems. For example, when we say "graph paper," we almost always mean paper ruled in squares suitable for easy handling of Cartesian graphing.

POLAR COORDINATES. Many specific problems require specific coordinate systems. The Cartesian coordinates are best suited for rectilinear problems, but not for problems involving circles; they are best handled by *polar coordinates*. In this system a position is determined by its distance (r) from the origin and the angle θ between r and the horizontal axis, as illustrated in Fig. 6-4.

It is often important to convert Cartesian coordinates into the equivalent polar coordinates and vice versa. With respect to a point defined by x and y, this is done by formulas 6-1 and 6-3: $r = \sqrt{x^2 + y^2}$ and $\tan \theta = {}^y/_x$. The conversion from polar to Cartesian coordinates can readily be derived. Consider point P_1 in Fig. 6-4. A vertical line from P_1 to the x-axis, the x-axis itself,

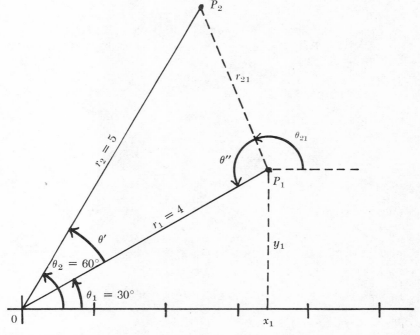

Fig. 6-4. Polar coordinates. Two points, P_1 and P_2, are illustrated in polar coordinates; P_1 is located at $r_1 = 4$ and $\theta_1 = 30°$. P_2 is located at $r_2 = 5$ and $\theta_2 = 60°$.

and the line from the origin to P_1 define a right triangle. If we call the base of this triangle x_1 and the height y_1, the trigonometric ratios for the sine and cosine are written as follows:

$$\sin \theta_1 = \frac{y_1}{r_1}$$

$$\cos \theta_1 = \frac{x_1}{r_1}$$

These can be rewritten as follows:

$$\boxed{x_1 = r_1 \cos \theta_1}$$ Formula 6-4

$$\boxed{y_1 = r_1 \sin \theta_1}$$ Formula 6-5

Example 6-6. What are the Cartesian coordinates for the point P_1 of Fig. 6-4? Since $r_1 = 4$ and $\theta_1 = 30°$, the coordinates are (from formulas 6-4 and 6-5) $x_1 = 4 \cos 30° = 4\left(\frac{\sqrt{3}}{2}\right) = 2\sqrt{3} \cong 3.5$ and $y_1 = 4 \sin 30° = 4(\frac{1}{2}) = 2$.

Distance and angles with respect to the origin are obviously very simply found in polar coordinates. Distances and directions involving points other than the origin are much more difficult to find here than in the Cartesian system.

First, consider distances. In Fig. 6-4 we wish to find r_{21}. The origin and points P_1 and P_2 define a triangle with sides r_1, r_2, and r_{21}. The angle θ' is $\theta_2 - \theta_1$. The value of r_{21} can be found from the cosine law (p. 112):

$$r_{21} = \sqrt{r_1{}^2 + r_2{}^2 - 2r_1 r_2 \cos (\theta_2 - \theta_1)}$$

In Fig. 6-4, $r_1 = 4$, $r_2 = 5$, $\theta = 30°$, and $\theta_2 = 60°$. Thus

$$r_{21} = \sqrt{4^2 + 5^2 - 2 \times 4 \times 5 \cos 30°}$$

$$\cong \sqrt{16 + 25 - 40 \times 0.8660} = \sqrt{6.359} = 2.52$$

Once the distance r_{21} is found, the sine law (p. 110) can be applied to find the angles

$$\frac{\sin \theta'}{r_{21}} = \frac{\sin \theta''}{r_2} \text{ and } \theta_{21} = 180° + \theta_1 - \theta''$$

In the example of Fig. 6-4, $\sin \theta'' = r_2 \dfrac{\sin \theta'}{r_{21}} \cong 5 \times \dfrac{\frac{1}{2}}{2.52} = 0.99$, or $\theta'' \cong 97.5°$.

Thus $\theta_{21} = 180° + 30 - 97.5 = 112.5°$.

Both calculations are obviously much more involved than the corresponding Cartesian calculation. For this reason, some people prefer to convert the polar to Cartesian coordinates by formulas 6-4 and 6-5 and then calculate angles and distances in this system.

> **Example 6-7.** Calculate the numerical value of r_{21} of Fig. 6-4 by first converting the coordinates of P_1 and P_2 to Cartesian coordinates. Example 6-6 showed that $x_1 = 2\sqrt{3} \cong 3.5$ and $y_1 = 2$. In a similar way the coordinates of point P_2 can be shown to be $x_2 = 5/2 = 2.5$ and $y_2 = 5\sqrt{3}/2 \cong 4.3$. Thus from formula 6-2:
>
> $$r_{12} = \sqrt{(x_2 - x_1)^2 + (y_2 - y_1)^2} \cong \sqrt{(2.5 - 3.5)^2 + (4.3 - 2)^2} = 2.5$$

OTHER COORDINATE SYSTEMS. Although there are many other plane coordinate systems, we will only show the *bipolar coordinate system* (Fig. 6-5) in which the coordinates are a pair of angles.

Of the many three-dimensional systems, we will briefly mention three. The *three-dimensional Cartesian system* utilizes three linear coordinates, usually called x, y, and z. The z-axis is at right angles to the x and y axes. This is illustrated in Fig. 6-6. The distance (r) from the origin to a point (P), at position x, y, z can be shown to be equal to $\sqrt{x^2 + y^2 + z^2}$.

In extending polar coordinates to three dimensions, one can utilize *cylindrical coordinates* that add the z-axis to the r and θ of the polar coordinates. In this case, the three cylindrical coordinates are related to the three Cartesian coordinates as $r = \sqrt{x^2 + y^2}$, $\tan \theta = y/x$, and $z = z$. Or, the Cartesian coordinates are given as $x = r \cos \theta$, $y = r \sin \theta$, and $z = z$.

Two angles and one length are used to locate a point in the *spherical coordinate system*. The length is the distance from the origin to the point, usually designated by r, just as in the cylindrical system. However, these rs are not the same. The spherical coordinates are shown in Fig. 6-7. The polar angle θ is the angle between the x-axis and the projection in the x-y plane of the line

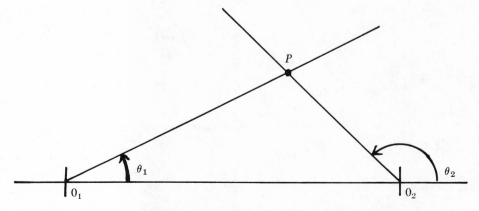

Fig. 6-5. Bipolar coordinates. In bipolar coordinates there are two origins a known distance apart. The coordinates of the point P are the angles at the two origins θ_1 and θ_2.

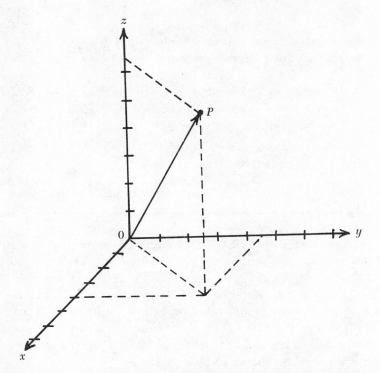

Fig. 6-6. Three-dimensional Cartesian coordinates. The conventional representation on a two-dimensional piece of paper is shown. The *y* and *z* axes are thought to lie in the plane of the paper; the *x*-axis projects out of the paper toward the reader. To clearly specify the point *P* in space, a projection must be shown. In this case the projection is on the *x-y* plane.

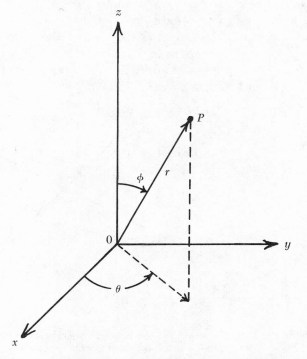

Fig. 6-7. The spherical coordinate system. A point (*P*) is defined in terms of its distance (*r*) from the origin and two angles, θ and ϕ.

from the origin to the point. The angle ϕ is formed by the z-axis and the line r. By finding appropriate right triangles it can be shown that:

$$r = \sqrt{x^2 + y^2 + z^2}$$

$$\tan \theta = {}^{y}/_{x}$$

$$\tan \phi = \frac{\sqrt{x^2 + y^2}}{z}$$

A full study of three-dimensional systems is not necessary here, but the basic terminology should be familiar.

TYPES OF GRAPHS

A graph in two dimensions is the representation of the functional relationships between two variables. In a Cartesian system, the vertical or y distance typically represents the dependent variable, whereas the horizontal or x distance represents the independent variable. For example, if we are to study the incidence of a certain cancer as a function of age, the incidence of the disease is the dependent variable and age the independent variable.

Just as there is no one coordinate system for all the problems of spatial representation, there is also no one way to draw all graphs. Most two-dimensional graphs are drawn in the Cartesian system and only rarely in polar coordinates.

There are several kinds of graphs. Data can be either experimental (empirical) or theoretical. The type of data to be displayed determines the type of graph to be used.

HISTOGRAMS, POINT GRAPHS, AND LINE GRAPHS. Experimental and, occasionally, theoretical data are often grouped according to the ranges of values of the independent variable. Such data may be plotted as *histograms,* as shown in Fig. 6-8. When age, time, patient height or weight, and similar

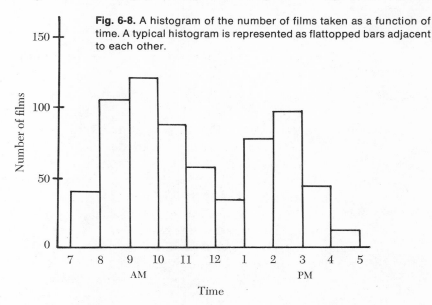

Fig. 6-8. A histogram of the number of films taken as a function of time. A typical histogram is represented as flattopped bars adjacent to each other.

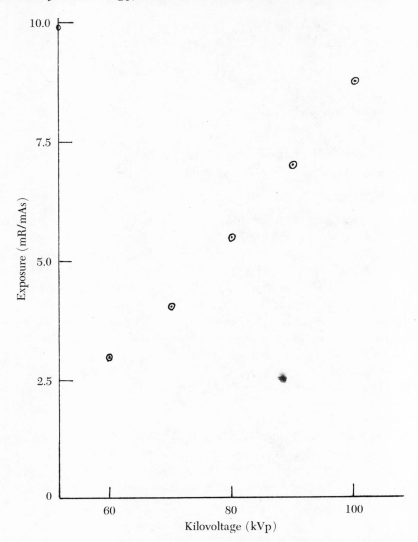

Fig. 6-9. A point graph of the exposure in mR/mAs as a function of the kilovoltage 100 cm from a typical radiographic unit.

quantities are the independent variable, this is often the best representation.

Frequently it is not convenient to measure the dependent variable for all values of the independent variable. For example, we know that the radiation output of an x-ray unit will vary with the peak voltage (kVp) across the x-ray tube. It is not practical to measure the output for all the kVp settings, but rather for selected values only, such as every 10 kVp. Since here we have only a sample of all the data possible, the results are best represented by a point for each sample. A *point graph* is shown in Fig. 6-9.

If our data express a continuous functional relationship, their graph should be continuous. This implies a theoretical origin. The theory may be conceived

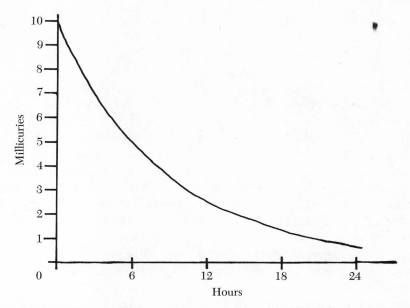

Fig. 6-10. A line graph of the amount of ^{99m}Tc activity remaining (starting with 10 mCi) as a function of time. This is a theoretical curve based on the law of exponential decay.

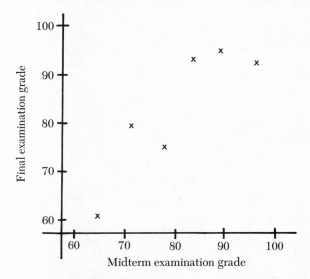

Fig. 6-11. A scatter diagram. Each point represents one individual.

of as a projection of *all* values of the independent variable. These would then form a series of very closely packed points that collectively constitute a line. A *line graph* is shown in Fig. 6-10. The point graph can be considered the graphic representation of a table; the line graph is the graphic representation of an algebraic function.

Another way of handling experimental relationships between two variables is to sample both simultaneously. For example, a height-weight study of humans could be carried out in which height is one variable and the weight is the other. Each individual height and weight measured would be entered as a point on a graph. The result of a series of such measurements would be a *scatter diagram*, as shown in Fig. 6-11. If there is a relationship of some sort between the variables, the scatter diagram will exhibit a geometric pattern. Otherwise, the result will be a random distribution of the points.

INTERPRETATION OF GRAPHS. All graphs are intended to represent a relationship between variables. A histogram (Fig. 6-8) shows the values of a dependent variable for increments of the independent variable. A point graph (Fig. 6-9) shows the relationship between dependent and independent variables for only a selected set of independent variable values. It will yield a table with as many pairs of entries as there are points on the graph. The line graph (Fig. 6-10) shows the relationship between *all* values of the independent and dependent variables for a given range. The line graph can be read as a table or, at least in principle, as a function.

The reading of a single point is essentially the same on any type of graph. Our examples will utilize Fig. 6-12, which is a line graph of the percent depth dose P, of a ^{60}Co beam. The curve can be considered as the relationship between P and the depth d. That is, the y coordinate of a point on the curve represents the value of P for the given value of d on the x coordinate. To read the graph for a specific value of d, a vertical line is drawn from that value on the x-axis to the curve and a horizontal line from the point of intersection to the y-axis. The value of P can then be read off the scale given on the y-axis.

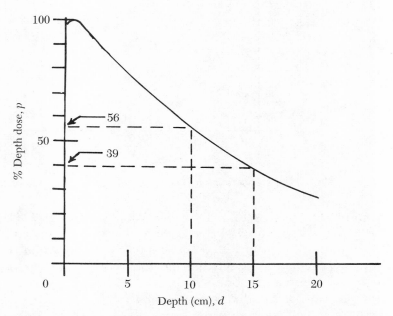

Fig. 6-12. The percent depth dose (P) for a ^{60}Co beam (entrance size 10 × 10 cm, source to skin distance 80 cm). The dotted lines are used to find P for d = 10 and d = 15.

For example, for $d = 10, P = 56$. On graph paper, it is often unnecessary to draw these lines.

> **Example 6-8.** Find the value of P for $d = 15$ cm in Fig. 6-12. The lines needed are shown in the figure. The result is $P = 39$.

> **Example 6-9.** Find the depth (d) for a percent depth dose of 75% in Fig. 6-12. If a horizontal line (not shown) is drawn from the value of P to the curve and a vertical line is dropped from the intersection to the horizontal axis, the value of d can be read off this axis; it is about 5.7 cm.

In point graphs we can only choose those values of the independent (x) variable for which a point is given. For an intermediate point, interpolation may be a possibility (see discussion of graphs of empirical data, p. 141).

> **Example 6-10.** For which values of kilovoltage can we obtain an exposure value in Fig. 6-9? There are five values represented by the five points. If we drop verticals from each point to the horizontal axis, we can read off their values: 60, 70, 80, 90, and 100 kVp.

> **Example 6-11.** What is the value of the exposure at 70 kVp in Fig. 6-9? We draw a line from the 70 kVp point perpendicular to the vertical axis. With this line (not shown) it can be seen that the exposure is about 4.1 mR/mAs.

Reading a graph does present certain problems of accuracy. Although even full-page graphs (about 20 cm high) are drawn with different degrees of care, they can rarely be read to greater accuracy than about 1 mm. An accuracy of better than 0.5% $\left(\dfrac{0.1}{20}\right)$ of the full scale amount is therefore unlikely. For smaller graphs it will be even less. In general, it is reasonable to assume an accuracy of about 1%.

Experimental data have certain inherent uncertainties. The statistical interpretation of this uncertainty will be considered in Chapter 9.

The *line graph*, exhibiting a *smooth curve*, that is, without discontinuities or sudden changes in the slope, is the bridge between algebra and geometry. It can be obtained from an algebraic function and is very useful in investigating those functions that give a good fit to experimental data.

Graphing a function. Any function can be converted to a table consisting of values of the dependent variable for selected values of the independent variable. In deriving a graph from a function we are free to select as many values of the independent variable as we wish, provided they are within the range for which the function was formulated. All points representing these values lie on

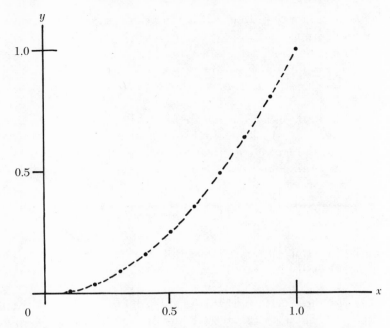

Fig. 6-13. Graph of the function $y = x^2$. The dots represent values that have been calculated for $x = 0.1, 0.2$, etc.

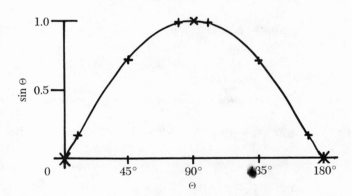

Fig. 6-14. The graph of sin θ for $0 \leq \theta \leq 180°$. The values for $\theta = 0, 90$, and 180 degrees (the Xs) are not enough to give the entire shape of the graph. With additional points at 10, 45, 80, 100, 135, and 170 degrees (the +s), the full shape becomes obvious.

a curve. If enough of them are plotted, the shape of the curve becomes clear. For example, the function $y = x^2$ can be solved for $x = 0, 0.1, 0.2, \ldots, 0.9, 1.0$. The results are $y = 0, 0.01, 0.04, \ldots, 0.81, 1.0$. These can be plotted as shown in Fig. 6-13. In this case the smooth curve *must* run exactly through all the points. If we are not certain of the curve shape, we can plot more points.

Example 6-12. Plot the curve for sin θ for values of θ from 0 to 180 degrees (0 to π in radians). First we find sin θ for $\theta = 0, 90$, and 180 degrees. We plot them as the x's in Fig. 6-14. But they are not adequate to determine the shape of a smooth curve. We need points near these three and some intermediate ones. The points for 10, 45, 80, 100, 135, and 170 degrees are shown as plus signs in the figure. With these points the smooth shape can be found.

Slope and tangent. One of the important parameters in a straight line graph (Fig. 6-15) is the *slope*. It can be defined in two ways. One is the angle θ between the line and the x-axis, which may vary from -90 to $+90$ degrees. The slope can also be expressed as the ratio of the "rise" over the "run." To obtain this ratio two convenient points on the graph are chosen and a right triangle is drawn as shown in the figure. The slope (m) is equal to the ratio of the height of the triangle (Δy) to its base (Δx). Obviously this ratio is also the tangent of the angle θ, hence:

$$m = \frac{\Delta y}{\Delta x} = \tan \theta \qquad\qquad \text{Formula 6-6}$$

Delta is used to represent "the change in." If we designate the two points on the graph as x_1, y_1, and x_2, y_2 then $\Delta x = x_2 - x_1$ and $\Delta y = y_2 - y_1$. The final amount is equal to the initial amount plus the amount of the change. If we had chosen other points on the curve, Δx and Δy would have been different, but the ratio $\left(\frac{\Delta x}{\Delta y}\right)$ would have been the same.

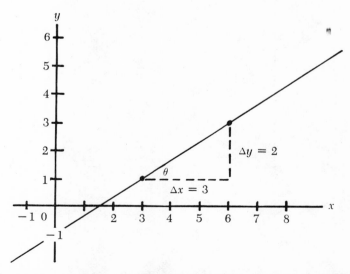

Fig. 6-15. A graph of straight line passing through two points. The straight line is characterized by the two *intercepts* (the intersection between the line and the two axes) and the slope. Here the x and y intercepts are $+1.5$ and -1. The slope (m) is equal to $\dfrac{\Delta y}{\Delta x}$; here $m = \frac{2}{3}$.

Example 6-13. What is the slope m of the straight line in Fig. 6-15? At the lower point on the curve in the figure, $x_1 = 3, y_1 = 1$. At the upper point, $x_2 = 6$, $y_2 = 3$. Thus $\Delta x = 3$ and $\Delta y = 2$, or $m = \frac{2}{3}$.

Example 6-14. Calculate the slope using the points of interception of this straight line with the axes $x_1 = 0, y_1 = -1$, and $x_2 = 1.5, y_2 = 0$. Here $\Delta x = 1.5 - 0 = 1.5, \Delta y = 0 - (-1) = 1$; therefore $m = \dfrac{\Delta y}{\Delta x} = \frac{1}{1.5} = \frac{2}{3}$.

If a straight line goes upward to the right (as in Fig. 6-15), the slope is positive. If the straight line is horizontal, the slope is 0, since $\Delta y = 0$. If the line goes down to the right, the slope is negative. The steeper the slope, the greater the magnitude.

For the curves that are not straight lines, the slope can also be defined, but there is no longer a single value. Consider the curve $y = x^2$ shown in Fig. 6-16. Two straight lines are drawn through the point $x = \frac{1}{4}, y = \frac{1}{4}$; for any point there is an infinity of such lines. The line that passes through the points $x = 0, y = 0$ and $x = \frac{1}{2}, y = \frac{1}{4}$ is said to have the *average slope* from $x = 0$ to $x =$

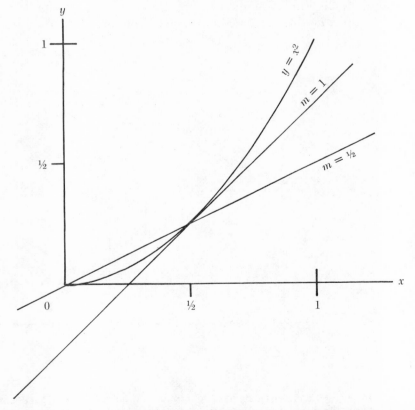

Fig. 6-16. A curve ($y = x^2$) passing through the point $x = \frac{1}{2}, y = \frac{1}{4}$. Two of the many possible straight lines passing through the point are shown. Their slope values (m) are $\frac{1}{2}$ and 1. The line with $m = 1$ is the tangent line.

$\frac{1}{2}$. An average slope is determined by using formula 6-6, in this case

$$m = \frac{\Delta y}{\Delta x} = \frac{(y_2 - y_1)}{(x_2 - x_1)} = \frac{1/4}{1/2} = \frac{1}{2}.$$

> **Example 6-15.** What is the average slope between $x = 0$ and $x = 1$
> for the curve $y = x^2$? At $x = 0$, $y = 0$ and at $x = 1$, $y = 1$; thus
> $$m = \frac{\Delta y}{\Delta x} = \frac{(1 - 0)}{(1 - 0)} = \frac{1}{1} = 1.$$

For a point on a smooth curve there is one and only one straight line that can go through the point and be exactly parallel to the curve at the point. For the point $x = \frac{1}{2}$, $y = \frac{1}{4}$ on the curve $y = x^2$ this line has a slope of 1. This line is called the *tangent line* at that point. Usually the tangent line does not cross the curve at the point of tangency.

Functional forms. As we have seen, a straight line can be characterized completely by two of the following parameters: the slope m, the x intercept, and the y intercept. When two of these are known, the third can be found (see example 6-14). Here we are interested in finding the functional form of a specific straight line, such as the one shown in Fig. 6-17. To do so, we can use the definition of the slope and its value, and a known point such as one of the intercepts. In the process we will define an additional point, labeled P in the figure, situated anywhere on the line. Using the y intercept as one of the points, $x_2 = 0$, $y_2 = 4$; $x_1 = x$, $y_1 = y$ and $m = -\frac{1}{2}$, then $\frac{\Delta y}{\Delta x} = \frac{4 - y}{0 - x} = -\frac{1}{2}$; multiplying by $-x$, we obtain $4 - y = +\frac{1}{2}x$. Solving this for y yields the

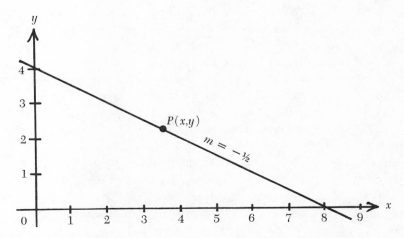

Fig. 6-17. A graph of a straight line. The line has the functional form $y = 4 - \frac{1}{2}x$.

equation $y = 4 - \frac{1}{2}x$. Since P could be located at any place on the line, this equation must represent the functional form for any point on the line. The general functional form for any straight line is:

$$y = y_0 + mx \hspace{4cm} \text{Formula 6-7}$$

where the variable y_0 is the y intercept and m is the slope. We now understand why the functional form $y = A + Bx$ is called "linear"—because it corresponds to a straight line graph.

> **Example 6-16.** What is the equation for the straight line of Fig. 6-15? Here the value of the slope m is $\frac{2}{3}$ and of the y intercept is -1. The equation for the line is $y = -1 + \frac{2x}{3}$.

To find the equation of a straight line it is not always necessary that the y intercept be known. Rather, we can use the definition of the slope in the manner used in deriving formula 6-7.

> **Example 6-17.** Use the slope ($m = -\frac{1}{2}$) and the x intercept ($x_1 = 8$, $y_1 = 0$) to derive the equation of the line in Fig. 6-17. The point P corresponds to $x_2 = x$, $y_2 = y$. The defining equation for the slope can be written as $\dfrac{y_2 - y_1}{x_2 - x_1} = m$, or $\dfrac{y - 0}{x - 8} = -\frac{1}{2}$. Multiplying both sides by $x - 8$ yields $y - 0 = -\frac{1}{2}(x - 8)$, or $y = 4 - \frac{1}{2}x$ as before.

The functional form of the straight line is easily found because its slope does not change.

The constant function $y = A$ can be considered as a special case of formula 6-7 where the straight line has a slope of zero. This means that the graph of a constant function is a horizontal straight line.

It is difficult to be precise about the graphs of nonlinear functions without using calculus. Logarithms (Chapter 8) permit modification of several functions to a linear form. Here we will simply follow a descriptive course with some of the principal features.

If we write out a function having one or more constants and then plot the graph for various values of *one* of the constants, a family of curves is obtained, as shown for $y = ax^2$ in Fig. 6-18.

The most frequently used "power" form of a function is the quadratic form involving x^2. Fig. 6-18 shows the family of curves for the simplest form of this curve. For a given value of the constant A in $y = Ax^2$, the curve has a ∪ shape that is symmetrical about the y-axis, because $(-x)^2 = x^2$ and is always positive. If the constant A is positive, the curve "opens" upward. If A is negative, the curve "opens" downward. Replacing A with $-A$ will produce the mirror image curve as reflected through the x-axis. These curves are known as *parabolas*.

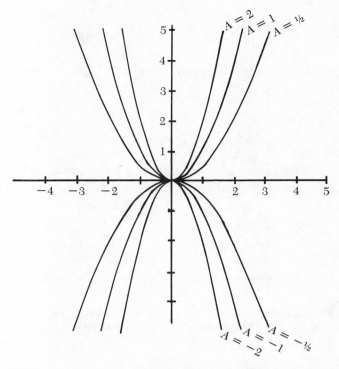

Fig. 6-18. A family of parabolas, $y = Ax^2$, passing through the origin. The parabolas are symmetrical about the y-axis.

The function $y = C + Ax^2$ is also a parabola symmetrical about the y-axis and opening upward if $A > 0$. However, the y intercept for this curve is not the origin but $y = C$. The function $y = C + Bx + Ax^2$ is also a parabola opening upward or downward, depending on the sign of A. The y intercept is C, but the minimum point is not on the y-axis if $B \neq 0$ and the curve is symmetrical about a vertical line other than the y-axis.

The parabola is a very important curve both for the representation of the common quadratic functions (an example is the radiation output of an x-ray machine as function of kVp) and for certain spatial problems.

Another group of functions are the inverse powers; particularly the inverse $(y = 1/x = x^{-1})$ and the inverse square $(y = 1/x^2 = x^{-2})$. Both are plotted for positive values of x in Fig. 6-19. The shape of the inverse function is called a *hyperbola*. Both of these functions are very important in radiology; the relationship between the ionization chamber pressure correction factor and the pressure $(C_P = {}^{760}/_P)$ is one example of an inverse function. The inverse square function is important for determining the radiation intensity from a point source, as discussed in Chapter 4.

Trigonometric functions. The graph of the *trigonometric function* $y = \sin x$ is shown in Fig. 6-20; it has the characteristic wave shape. The simplest waves in physics are "sine waves." They are very important in the analysis of *periodic* systems, those that return to essentially the same position at regular

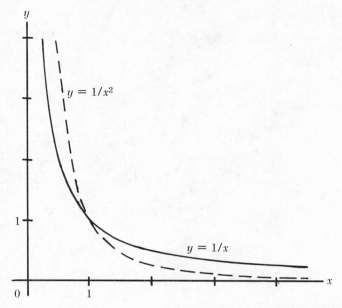

Fig. 6-19. Graphic representation of an inverse function ($y = 1/x$) and an inverse square function ($y = 1/x^2$). The shape of the inverse function $y = 1/x$ is a hyperbola.

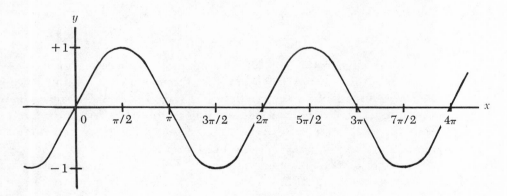

Fig. 6-20. Graph of a trigonometric function ($y = \sin x$). Usually, x is expressed in radians as shown. If it is written $y = \sin \theta$, the angle is usually expressed in degrees.

intervals. Many physical and biological systems approximate periodicity. For example, AC electricity and synchronized cell populations in the "cell cycle" are two essentially periodic systems.

The sine wave is characterized by three distinct elements: amplitude, wavelength, and phase. The *wavelength* is the distance between the tops of two successive waves. In Fig. 6-20, the wavelength is 2π. The wave oscillates above and below the x-axis. The maximum displacement from the x-axis is called the *amplitude*. In Fig. 6-20 the amplitude is 1.0.

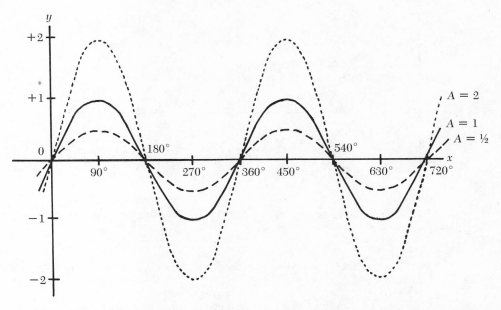

Fig. 6-21. A family of curves having the same wavelength but different amplitudes ($y = A \sin x$). The constant A is the amplitude.

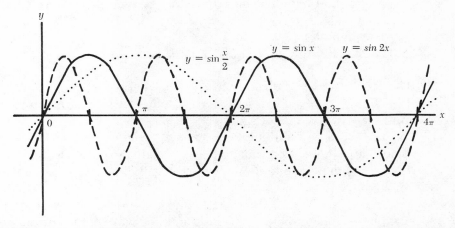

Fig. 6-22. Graph of the function $y = A \sin Kx$, where $A = 1$ and $K = \frac{1}{2}$, 1, and 2. The amplitudes of these waves are the same, but the wavelengths are different.

The sine wave function can be written with two constants (A and k) in the form $y = A \sin kx$. From the examples in Fig. 6-21 it can be seen that the constant A corresponds to the amplitude (the maximum displacement of the wave from the x-axis).

If the value of k changes and A remains constant, the amplitude of the wave remains the same but the wavelength changes. This is shown in Fig. 6-22. The relationship between k and the wavelength (λ) is

$$\lambda = \frac{2\pi}{k}$$

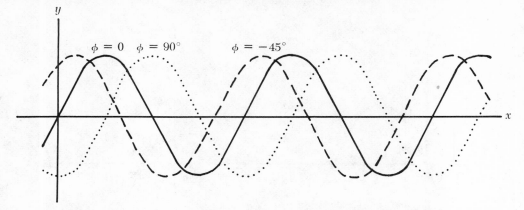

Fig. 6-23. Sine waves of different phases (ϕ) but with the same amplitude and wavelength. The general form of these curves is $y = \sin(x - \phi)$.

For this reason the equation for a sine wave is sometimes written as follows:

$$y = A \sin \frac{2\pi x}{\lambda}$$

Example 6-18. What is the amplitude and wavelength of the wave $y = \frac{3}{2} \sin 2\pi x$? The amplitude can be read directly as $\frac{3}{2}$: the wavelength is $\lambda = \frac{2\pi}{k} = 2\pi(\frac{1}{k})$. Since $k = 2\pi$, the amplitude is $\frac{3}{2}$ and the wavelength is 1.0.

The third parameter is called the *phase*. The general form can be written as $y = A \sin(\frac{2\pi x}{\lambda} - \phi)$, where ϕ is a constant, the "phase angle." In all previous examples $\phi = 0$.

In Fig. 6-23, sine waves of the same wavelength and amplitude but differing phases are shown. For a positive phase angle the entire curve is shifted by the amount of the angle to the left; for a negative phase angle, the shift is to the right.

The term "phase" is also part of the AC electrical vocabulary. Here, "single phase" means that there is only one sine wave of the current or voltage in the supply. A "three-phase" system has three waves on three different wires; the waves are $\frac{2\pi}{3}$, or 120 degrees, out of phase with each other.

Graphic solution of equations. Linear equations and some others can be solved algebraically as described in Chapter 3. Sometimes it is more convenient to solve them graphically.

The general form of an equation can be written as follows:

$$f(x) = g(x)$$

Unless these two expressions are essentially the same, there is a limited set of values (solutions) for x that satisfy this relationship. The *graphic solutions* are found by plotting $y = f(x)$ and $y = g(x)$ as line graphs. Any solutions must lie on both of the lines, that is, the solutions occur where the lines cross.

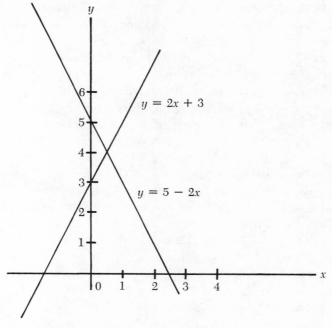

Fig. 6-24. The solution of the equation $2x + 3 = 5 - 2x$. The two straight lines $y = 2x + 3$ and $y = 5 - 2x$ are plotted. Their intersection at $x = \frac{1}{2}$ (and $y = 4$) represents the solution.

Example 6-19. Solve the equation $2x + 3 = 5 - 2x$. First $y = 3 + 2x$ and $y = 5 - 2x$ are plotted (Fig. 6-24). They cross at $x = \frac{1}{2}$, $y = 4$. The y intersection is not important here; the solution is $x = \frac{1}{2}$.

If the expressions are linear, as in the preceding example, the graphs will be straight lines. Straight lines can only intersect at one point. If the functions are not linear, there is no guarantee of a single solution. There may be several solutions or no solution at all. For many equations, graphic solutions are an easy first step, but due to the inherent limitations on reading graphs, other methods may be needed for a more precise determination.

GRAPHS OF EMPIRICAL DATA

Data obtained from experimental measurements (empirical data) are often presented in graphic form to illustrate a more or less precise relationship between the variables in an experiment or data sample. Sometimes the experiment closely approximates the situation for which these data are to be used. For example, if we measure radiation output for 100 mAs at 70, 80, and 100 kVp at a distance of 100 cm from a radiographic unit, we roughly approximate the actual use of the equipment in many common situations. However, if we consider it impractical to make all our measurements at or near the anticipated use parameters, we may wish to extract a theoretical result, probably in functional form.

CHOICE OF FORM. There are several possibilities for presenting empirical data. The form to be used depends primarily on the type of data. For example, we prefer to use histograms to show categories such as 10-year intervals in a patient census. Numerical intervals need not always be equal. In particular, "exciting" regions may be broken into smaller intervals than "quiet" ones. For example, since human mortality statistics as a function of age show the highest figures in the early and late years, these should have narrower intervals than the intervening years. Similarly, if departmental statistics are being plotted by time, narrower intervals might be used for periods when new facilities, equipment, or procedures are introduced.

Whereas a histogram implies that the measurements taken represent the entire quantity within a category, a substantial sampling, or at least a legitimate average, in many instances it is easier to take just a sample for a specific value of the independent variable. Such instances are the output of an x-ray machine for specific kilovolt values with fixed milliamperage or the activity of a radioactive sample at specific times. Data such as these should be plotted as a point graph where the x-coordinates of the dots represent the independent variable and the y-coordinates represent the results of our measurements. Fig. 6-9 is an example of such a graph.

> **Example 6-20.** In a study of calibration accuracy 20 teletherapy machines were investigated; 6 machines were found to be within 1% of the standard, 7 between 1% and 2%, etc. Should these data be plotted as a histogram or as a point graph? Since the data are grouped by categories, they should be plotted as a histogram.

BEST FIT LINES. Experimental data often show a fairly clear-cut trend. If we took enough "perfect" measurements, we might expect the resulting points to form a single, smooth line. However, in the typical study, the points may approximate a smooth line, but they do not lie exactly on such a line because of experimental error or uncertainty. Nevertheless, it is the underlying line we are interested in and not the experimental points themselves. In some instances we may want to carry this one step further and obtain the algebraic form of the relationship. To obtain a well-fitting line, we must first consider what sort of line we wish to use. The more crooked a line is, the better we can fit it to the data points. With a line with sharp bends we can achieve a perfect fit if there are about as many bends as data points (Fig. 6-25). Normally we do not expect the underlying theory to have many sudden changes that would lead to a *broken line*. Whereas a broken line fit may make a perfect fit to a particular set of experimental data, it will probably not be a particularly good fit for another data set. In addition, we can also achieve an exact fit with a *smooth line* provided the line contains enough bends.

If we do not accept numerous breaks or bends in our lines, the fit will not be perfect. In this case a *good fit* is one that passes near enough (usually within

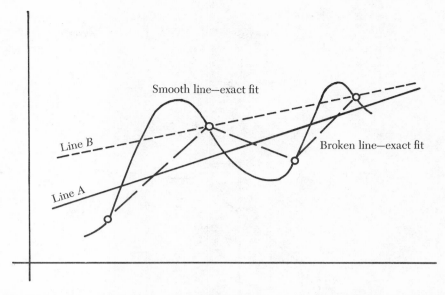

Fig. 6-25. Several fits to four data points. A perfect fit can be obtained with a broken line drawn from point to point or by various smooth curves that contain sufficient bends. There are other smooth fits that do not go through some of the points. Straight lines *A* and *B* are examples. Line *A* is a better fit than line *B*.

the experimental error) to the data points. Two straight lines are shown in Fig. 6-25. Line A is a much better fit than line B.

Probably the most popular technique of line fitting is the "eyeball" fit. In this case we simply draw the line that appears to us to give the best fit. This will be a line that runs close to almost all the points and has about as many points above the line as below.

If we have data that fall almost in a straight line, there is no problem with an eyeball fit. As the points scatter farther from a straight line the eyeball fit becomes more unreliable. It also becomes harder to justify the choice of one line over another. Such a situation is illustrated in Fig. 6-26, where two rather different eyeball fits are shown. Here it is best to rely on a mathematically derived fit rather than one in which subjective idiosyncrasies enter.

The most common mathematical method of fit is the method of *least squares*, which minimizes the sum of the squares of the vertical distances from all points to the line. The significance of this approach and the derivation of the following formulation can be found in standard texts; we will concentrate on the use of this fitting technique.

The graphed data (Fig. 6-26) can be considered as a series of points represented as paired coordinates: (x_1, y_1), (x_2, y_2), and so on. If the data are in the form of a histogram of equal intervals, the value for each interval of the independent variable is equated with the center of the interval. For unequal intervals the data should be subdivided into equal intervals. The data then consist of the value pairs x_i, y_i for the ith point. With these values we can define various sums (n points are assumed).

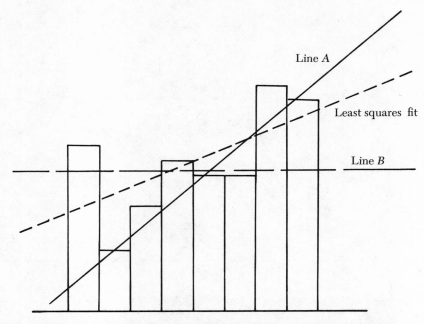

Fig. 6-26. Two straight-line "eyeball" fits (lines *A* and *B*) drawn by two different people to scattered data. Clearly, there is a great difference in the interpretation of the experimental results. The least squares fit is a widely accepted approach.

$$S_x = x_1 + x_2 + x_3 + \ldots \ldots \ldots \ldots \ldots \ldots +x_n$$
$$S_y = y_1 + y_2 + y_3 + \ldots \ldots \ldots \ldots \ldots \ldots +y_n$$
$$S_{xx} = x_1^2 + x_2^2 + x_3^2 + \ldots \ldots \ldots \ldots \ldots +x_n^2$$
$$S_{xy} = x_1 y_1 + x_2 y_2 + x_3 y_3 + \ldots \ldots \ldots \ldots +x_n y_n$$

The formula of a straight line was given earlier (formula 6-7). It is represented here as follows:

$$y = y_0 + mx$$

For the best fit straight line, the constants appearing in this formula are given by the two formulas:

$$y_0 = \frac{S_y S_{xx} - S_{xy} S_x}{n S_{xx} - (S_x)^2} \qquad \text{Formula 6-8}$$

$$m = \frac{n S_{xy} - S_x S_y}{n S_{xx} - (S_x)^2} \qquad \text{Formula 6-9}$$

Example 6-21. Find the least squares fit line for the three points $(x_1 = 1, y_1 = 3)$, $(x_2 = 2, y_2 = 3)$, and $(x = 3, y = 1)$. The sums are:

$S_x = 1 + 2 + 3 = 6$
$S_y = 3 + 3 + 1 = 7$
$S_{xx} = 1^2 + 2^2 + 3^2 = 1 + 4 + 9 = 14$
$S_{xy} = 1 \cdot 3 + 2 \cdot 3 + 3 \cdot 1 = 3 + 6 + 3 = 12$

In this case $y_0 = \dfrac{(7 \cdot 14 - 12 \cdot 6)}{(3 \cdot 14 - 6^2)} = \dfrac{26}{6} \cong 4.33,$

and $m \cong \dfrac{(3 \cdot 12 - 6 \cdot 7)}{(3 \cdot 14 - 6^2)} = \dfrac{-6}{6} = -1.0.$

In formulas 6-8 and 6-9 the denominators are the same; this can be used to speed calculations.

Two items deserve brief mention here: First, fitting formulas analogous to formulas 6-8 and 6-9 exist for certain curved lines, and second, "goodness of fit" of any particular line is amenable to mathematical evaluation. For straight lines this is frequently calculated using the coefficient of correlation. This coefficient is 1 if all the data lie on a straight line and is about 0.4 or less for completely random data exhibiting no trend.

Smoothing, interpolation, and extrapolation. Sometimes we recognize the presence of fluctuations inherent in experimental data, but are interested in a fluctuation-free average value. This average can often be approximated by a well-fitting smooth line. In many experimental situations *smoothing* is a valuable technique.

Fitted lines can also be used to evaluate the function for a point between two experimental or theoretical points. The process is called *interpolation* and is described in Chapter 11.

If a fitted line is extended beyond a series of points, we speak of *extrapolation*. Both interpolated and extrapolated values are approximations. The greater the distance from a known value the greater the potential error in the approximation. The uncertainty in extrapolated values is much greater than in interpolated values.

NOMOGRAMS. A *nomogram* is a graphic representation of mathematical relations used as a tool for computation. A nomogram for finding the average of two numbers is shown in Fig. 6-27.

> **Example 6-22.** Use Fig. 6-27 to find the average of 3.5 and 5.5. We place a ruler in such a way that it crosses the *A* scale of the Fig. at 3.5 and the *B* scale at 5.5. The average is read from the "average" scale and is found to be 4.5.

This is a trivial operation, used here simply as an illustration. In typical nomograms, lines are drawn (or a straight edge is used) between two scales to locate a point on a third scale. With parallel scales the operation is basically addition or subtraction. This can be modified to yield multiplication or division by using logarithmic scales.

Nomograms do not have any inherent magic. The functions they represent could be expressed in other ways. Any error or approximation in the underly-

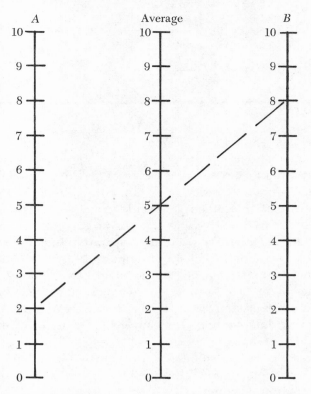

Fig. 6-27. A nomogram for obtaining averages. A straight line drawn from the value of A to the value of B will cross the center line at the average value of A and B. The example of the average of 2 and 8 is shown.

ing theory or model will result in less than perfect results in the use of the nomogram. Furthermore, any nomogram suffers from the usual inaccuracies of graphs, that is, a reading error of approximately 1% of full scale for normal-sized figures that are carefully drawn. The advent of electronic calculators has greatly reduced the use of nomograms.

CHAPTER REVIEW

1. What are the advantages of graphic representation of a function compared with algebraic representation?
2. What are the coordinates required to specify a point in the Cartesian coordinate system? In the polar system?
3. Can all points specified in the Cartesian system be specified in the polar system? Is the converse true?
4. What are the distinctive properties of a histogram? A point graph? A line graph? A scatter diagram?
5. Which types of graphs are most suitable for theoretical data?
6. How is a line graph read?
7. How is "slope" defined?
8. What do "Δx" and "Δy" mean in words?
9. What is the algebraic function of a straight line?
10. Define the terms "amplitude," "wave-

length," and "phase" with respect to a graph of the function sin θ.

11. Describe the graphic method of obtaining solutions to equations.
12. What is meant by a "best fit" function?
13. What is a nomogram?

PROBLEMS

Problems paralleling chapter examples

1. **(6-2)** What is the distance from the origin to point Q in Fig. 6-2?
2. **(6-3)** What is the distance between the points (3,2) and (2,3)?
3. **(6-4)** What is the angle between the line from the origin to point (3,6) and the x-axis?
4. **(6-5)** What is the distance between points (−2,2) and (−1,−1)?
5. **(6-6)** What are the Cartesian coordinates of point $r = 10$, $\theta = 40°$?
6. **(6-8)** Find the value of P for $d = 5$ cm in Fig. 6-12.
7. **(6-9)** At what depth does P have a value of 50% in Fig. 6-12?
8. **(6-11)** What is the value of the output at 90 kVp for the radiographic unit of Fig. 6-9?
9. **(6-12)** Plot the function $y = \tan \theta$ for θ between 0° and 75°.
10. **(6-13)** What is the slope of the straight line that could be drawn from P to Q in Fig. 6-2?
11. **(6-19)** Use graphic methods to find the two solutions to the equation $4x = x^2$.

Problems related to this chapter

12. What is the distance from the origin to point (4,6)?
13. What is the distance from point (2,−1) to point (1,3)?
14. What are the polar coordinates of point (7,17)?
15. Find the Cartesian coordinates of the point represented in polar coordinates by $r = 10$, $\theta = 45°$.
16. For a certain department the number of work days per month for a certain year was:

Janurary	1,090	July	826
February	983	August	915
March	1,102	September	1,047
April	1,037	October	1,108
May	984	November	1,095
June	883	December	1,004

Plot these data on graph paper as a histogram.

17. The temperature of the developer in a certain processor is measured at 7:30 AM each day. The results for a week were:

Monday	94.3	Friday	95.1
Tuesday	95.2	Saturday	95.3
Wednesday	94.9	Sunday	95.1
Thursday	94.6		

Plot these data as a point graph.

18. Plot the function $y = 1 - x^2$ for values of x between −2 and +2.
19. Fig. 6-28 shows the K-shell fluorescent yield as a function of atomic number. Find the fluorescent yield for the atomic numbers 7, 15, 50, and 100.
20. What are the slopes of the two lines in Fig. 6-24?
21. Use the method of least squares to find the best fit line for the data of problem 17. Use Monday as day 1, Tuesday as day 2, and so on, to give a numerical scale to the time.
22. The nomogram of Fig. 6-27 can be used to double a number. The technique is to draw a line through 0 on the A scale and through the number on the av scale. The

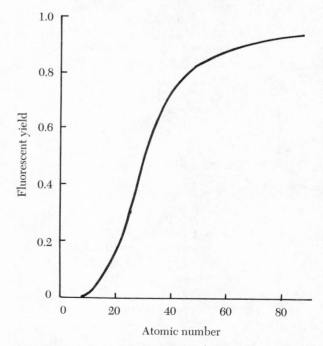

Fig. 6-28. Fluorescent yield for K-shell transitions as a function of atomic number.

result is read where this line crosses the *B* scale. Verify this method for doubling the numbers 1, 1.5, and 3. Why does this *not* work for 7 or −3?

Objective questions

23. A point is located 10 cm from the origin and at a polar angle of 30 degrees. The trigonometric ratios for 30 degrees are sin 30° = 0.5, cos 30° = 0.87, and tan 30° = 0.58. The *x* coordinate of this point is:
    a. 5
    b. 5.8
    c. 8.7
    d. 10
    e. 20

24. The distance between points *P* (*x* = 1, *y* = 3) and *Q* (*x* = 4, *y* = 0) is about:
    a. 1
    b. 2
    c. 3
    d. 4
    e. 5

25. The slope of a straight line is defined by the:
    a. ratio of the *x* intercept to *y* intercept
    b. ratio $\Delta y/\Delta x$
    c. sine of the angle between the line and the horizontal
    d. value of *y* when *x* = 1

26. A point is located at 2, 2. The distance from this point to the origin is _____ units.
    a. 2.0
    b. 2.8
    c. 4.0
    d. 3.5
    e. 3.9

27. The point 2, 2 has a polar angle of:
    a. 0 degrees
    b. 30 degrees
    c. 45 degrees
    d. 60 degrees
    e. 90 degrees

28. The most common coordinate system for graphs is:
    a. Cartesian
    b. cylindrical
    c. polar
    d. spherical
    e. transaxial

29. An algebraic function is properly graphed as a:
    a. scatter diagram
    b. line graph
    c. point graph
    d. histogram

30. The best fitting straight line is one that:
    a. minimizes the square of the deviation of all the points
    b. passes through all the most important points
    c. is mathematically exact
    d. passes through the maximum number of points

31. The function *y* = 4 + 6*x* will graph as a:
    a. straight line with positive slope
    b. straight line with zero slope
    c. straight line with negative slope
    d. parabola opening upward
    e. parabola opening downward

32. A point is located at *x* = 3, *y* = 3. The distance of this point from the origin is:
    a. $\sqrt{3}$
    b. $\sqrt{18}$
    c. 6
    d. 9
    e. 18

33. A point is located at *r* = 4 cm and θ = 90 degrees. The *x* and *y* coordinates of this point are:
    a. 4,0
    b. 2,2
    c. $2\sqrt{2}, 2\sqrt{2}$
    d. 1,3
    e. 0,4

34. The graph of the sine function can be described as:
    a. 1,3,4
    b. 2
    c. 5
    d. 1,4
    e. 3
    (1) a periodic function
    (2) monotonic increasing
    (3) a straight line
    (4) a wave
    (5) monotonic decreasing

35. Which of the following will graph as a straight line on regular graph paper?
    a. $y = x^2$
    b. $y = 2 + x$
    c. $y = 1/x$
    d. $y = e^{+2x}$
    e. $y = \log x$

CHAPTER 7

Powers and exponentials

The use of *powers* has already been demonstrated for squares, cubes, and other expressions. This concept can be extended in several important ways. The *exponential* formulation, discussed later in this chapter, is particularly useful in radiology, since photon attenuation, radioactive decay, light absorption, and certain other radiological results all follow exponential relationships.

LAWS OF EXPONENTS

The concept of powers provides a convenient notation for eliminating a variety of mathematical operations, especially those involving products, quotients, and roots.

MULTIPLICATION WITH EXPONENTS. Consider the product $3^2 \times 3^4$. In Chapter 1 we saw that powers multiply as $3^2 \times 3^4 = 3^{(2+4)} = 3^6$. This property can be verified for this example by expanding the powers and then counting the number of factors of 3. The expression 3^2 will contribute two factors and 3^4 will contribute four, for a total of 6. This property will hold even if the *base** is an algebraic variable or expression. Thus $x^2 \times x^3 = x^5$ and $(x + y)^4(x + y)^2 = (x + y)^6$. In general:

$$x^a \times x^b = x^{a+b}$$

Formula 7-1

Exponents can be added only if the bases are the same. For example, $2^3 \times 5^2$ can be written in other ways, but none of these would give a power of $3 + 2$, or 5. If more than one base is present in a product, each base can be handled separately, since the law of commutation holds. For example, $2^3 3^2 \times 2^4 3 = 2^3 2^4 3^2 3 = 2^{(3+4)} 3^{(2+1)} = 2^7 3^3$.

> **Example 7-1.** Simplify $(x^2yz^3)(x^3y^2z)$. This is equal to $x^2x^3yy^2z^3z = x^5y^3z^4$.

Formula 7-1 works for powers that are variables, expressions, fractions, or negative values. These will be considered in later sections of this chapter.

---

*In this context, the base is the number taken to the power specified. For example, 3 is the base in the expression 3^5.

DIVISION WITH EXPONENTS. Consider $\dfrac{2^4}{2^2}$. This is equal to $^{16}/_4 = 4 = 2^2$. In general:

$$x^n/x^m = x^{n-m} \qquad \text{Formula 7-2}$$

Example 7-2. Simplify $\dfrac{x^4y^7}{x^2y^3}$. By formula 7-2, $\dfrac{x^4}{x^2} = x^2$ and $\dfrac{y^7}{y^3} = y^4$. Thus $\dfrac{x^4y^7}{x^2y^3} = x^2y^4$.

Example 7-3. Simplify $\dfrac{6.0 \times 10^5}{4.0 \times 10^3}$. The division $\dfrac{6.0}{4.0}$ is simply 1.5; the powers of 10 are handled by formula 7-2 to give $\dfrac{10^5}{10^3} = 10^2$. Thus $\dfrac{6.0 \times 10^5}{4.0 \times 10^3} = 1.5 \times 10^2$.

Multiplication and division of powers can be carried out in a single step. For example, $\dfrac{3^5 \times 3^3}{3^4} = 3^{5+3-4} = 3^4$.

POWERS OF POWERS. In some instances we have to compute the *power of a power*. For example, $(x^3)^2$ is short for the product of $(x^3)(x^3)$. In the form $(A^k)^m$, the m implies m factors of the form A^k, for a combined power of $k \times m$ or:

$$\boxed{(A^k)^m = A^{km}} \qquad \text{Formula 7-3}$$

Example 7-4. Simplify $(3^4)^2$. This is equal to 3^8.

POWER OF A PRODUCT OR QUOTIENT. Consider the cube of the product ab, or $(ab)^3$. This is equal to $ababab$; utilizing commutation, the as and the bs can be grouped to give a^3b^3. In general:

$$\boxed{(ab)^n = a^nb^n} \qquad \text{Formula 7-4}$$

Example 7-5. One foot is equal to 12 inches; 1 inch is equal to 2.54 cm. Express 1 cubic foot in terms of centimeters using 12 and 2.54, but do not actually multiply. One foot is equal to 12×2.54 cm. One cubic foot is equal to $(12 \times 2.54)^3$ cm^3, or $12^3 \times 2.54^3$ cm^3.

Notice that *the power of a product is equal to the product of the power of the separate multiplicands.* If one of the multiplicands is a power, then Formulas 7-3 and 7-4 both apply. For example, $(xy^3)^2 = x^2y^6$. For the power of a quotient the situation is similar. The numerator and denominator are separately raised to the power:

$$\left(\frac{x}{y}\right)^k = \frac{x^k}{y^k}$$

Formula 7-5

Example 7-6. Express $\left(\frac{x^2}{y}\right)^3 \left(\frac{y}{x^2}\right)^2$ with a single power of x and y. These expand to $\left(\frac{x^6}{y^3}\right)\left(\frac{y^2}{x^4}\right)$, which simplifies to $\frac{x^2}{y}$.

ZERO AND NEGATIVE EXPONENTS. The concept of powers can be extended to include *zero and negative powers*. The extension is carried out in a manner consistent with the normal rules of algebra and the formulas developed in the preceding section of this chapter.

Zero powers. The *zero power* is most readily derived from formula 7-2:

$$\frac{x^n}{x^m} = x^{n-m}$$

If $n = m$, then $x^{n-m} = x^0$. In this case, the terms on the left of the equation become $\frac{x^m}{x^m}$; this is equal to 1. Thus:

$$x^0 = 1$$

Formula 7-6

for any value of x except $x = 0$ or $x = \infty$.

Example 7-7. What is e^0 (e is the base of the natural logarithm, approximately 2.72)? Formula 7-6 applies; e^0 is just 1.

Negative powers. Formula 7-2 has another extension. Consider the case of $m > n$, say, $m = 3$, $n = 1$. Formula 7-2 indicates that $\frac{x}{x^3} = x^{-2}$. Also $\frac{x}{x^3} = \frac{1}{x^2}$; this shows $x^{-2} = \frac{1}{x^2}$. The minus sign signifies that the power is in the denominator, or, in general terms:

$$a^{-n} = \frac{1}{a^n}$$

Formula 7-7

If a and n, in this formula, are both greater than 1, then $a^{-n} < 1$. For example, $2^{-3} = \frac{1}{2^3} = \frac{1}{8}$.

Example 7-8. The activity (A) of a radioactive sample of initial activity A_0 is $A = A_0(\frac{1}{2})^k$, where k is the number of half-lives to which the sample has been decaying. Use formula 7-7 to eliminate the fraction $\frac{1}{2}$. $(\frac{1}{2})^k = \frac{1}{2k} = 2^{-k}$. Thus the activity can be expressed as $A = A_o \, 2^{-k}$.

FRACTIONAL EXPONENTS. The powers considered so far have been integers, whether they are positive or negative. Formula 7-3 can be used for powers that are common fractions.

Significance of fractional exponents. Consider formula 7-3 for the special case where $k = \frac{1}{2}$ and $m = 2$. Then $(a^{\frac{1}{2}})^2 = a$. If the square of $a^{\frac{1}{2}}$ is a, then $a^{\frac{1}{2}}$ is the *square root* of a. For example, $4^{\frac{1}{2}} = 2$, $9^{\frac{1}{2}} = 3$, and so on. Thus the power $\frac{1}{2}$ is a convenient way to designate the square root.

> **Example 7-9.** Fractional exponents can be negative. What is the meaning of $16^{-\frac{1}{2}}$? The $\frac{1}{2}$ indicates the square root; the minus sign shows that it is in the denominator. Thus $16^{-\frac{1}{2}} = \frac{1}{4}$.

A cube root can be indicated by the fractional power $\frac{1}{3}$. In a similar way, all other roots can be indicated. What about expressions with an exponent that does not have 1 in the numerator? For example, what is the meaning of $x^{\frac{3}{4}}$? The $\frac{3}{4}$ is equal to $\frac{1}{4} \times 3$; the $\frac{1}{4}$ indicates the fourth root, whereas the 3 indicates a cube. Thus $16^{\frac{3}{4}}$ is equal to $(16^{\frac{1}{4}})^3 = 2^3$, or 8, since the fourth root of 16 is 2.

> **Example 7-10.** What is $27^{\frac{2}{3}}$? The cube root of 27 is 3 and $3^2 = 9$. Thus $27^{\frac{2}{3}} = 9$.

ROOTS AND RADICALS

The square root of a number is often indicated by the radical sign $\sqrt{}$ enclosing the number. Thus $\sqrt{5}$ is the square root of 5; it is equivalent to $5^{\frac{1}{2}}$. Other roots are indicated by the radical sign and the order of the root. Thus $\sqrt[3]{4}$ signifies the cube root of 4.

OPERATIONS WITH RADICALS. A *radical* is a root that cannot be expressed in terms of whole numbers, such as $\sqrt{2}$, $\sqrt[3]{9}$, and $\sqrt[5]{10}$, and its decimal representation is nonrepeating and nonterminating; for example, $\sqrt{2} = 1.414213562\ldots$ These properties make radicals difficult to manage mathematically.

Reduction to a lower order. The order of a radical is the order of the root involved; it is equal to the denominator of the power. Thus $\sqrt[5]{27} = 27^{\frac{1}{5}}$ is a fifth-order radical. If this order can be factored, it is possible to express the radical in a lower order. Consider $\sqrt[4]{9} = 9^{\frac{1}{4}}$. This is a fourth-order root; 4

can factor into 2×2. The expression $9^{1/4}$ can also be written as $\sqrt{\sqrt{9}} = (9^{1/2})^{1/2}$. Now $9^{1/2}$ is 3; therefore $9^{1/4} = 3^{1/2}$, or $\sqrt{3}$.

Example 7-11. Express the fourth root of 64 as a square root. The square root of 64 is 8; thus $\sqrt[4]{64} = \sqrt{8}$.

Multiplication and division of radicals. If radicals are of the same order, they are readily multiplied. This can be considered a reversal of formula 7-4, with the power now being fractional:

$$x^k y^k = (xy)^k$$

Formula 7-8A

or

$$\sqrt[p]{x}\ \sqrt[p]{y} = \sqrt[p]{xy}$$

Formula 7-8B

For example, $3^{1/2}\,2^{1/2} = (3 \times 2)^{1/2} = 6^{1/2}$.

If the radicals are not of the same order, an adjustment of the powers can be made. Multiplication of powers involves the addition of their exponents (formula 7-7); because these exponents can be fractions, a common denominator must be found. Consider, for example, the product $3^{1/2}5^{1/4}$. The common denominator for the exponents is 4, and thus the product can be written as $3^{2/4}5^{1/4}$, or $(3^2)^{1/4}5^{1/4}$. This can be multiplied by formula 7-8A to give $(3^2 5)^{1/4}$, or $45^{1/4}$.

Example 7-12. Express $2\sqrt{3}$ as a single number within the radical sign. We know that 2 is the square root of $2^2 = 4$. Thus $2\sqrt{3} = \sqrt{4}\sqrt{3} = \sqrt{4 \times 3} = \sqrt{12}$.

Division follows patterns similar to multiplication. It is based on formula 7-5, which can be rewritten as follows:

$$\frac{x^k}{y^k} = \left(\frac{x}{y}\right)^k$$

Formula 7-9A

$$\frac{\sqrt[p]{x}}{\sqrt[p]{y}} = \sqrt[p]{x/y}$$

Formula 7-9B

Simplification and rationalization of radicals. In the previous section, radicals were combined to single numbers. In some cases this process can be reversed to yield a more manageable form. This is called *simplification*. For example, $\sqrt{12} = 2\sqrt{3}$ (example 7-12). To carry this out in a routine manner, one looks for a factor of the base, here 12, that has a power equal to the order of the root. The number 12 factors to $2^2 3$.

Example 7-13. Simplify $\sqrt{4/45}$. The numerator factors to 2^2 and so $\sqrt{4} = 2$. The denominator factors to $3^2 5$; thus $\sqrt{45} = 3\sqrt{5}$. The combination of these is $\dfrac{2}{3\sqrt{5}}$.

Rationalization is the elimination of radicals from the denominator of a quotient. This is carried out by selective multiplication. For example, $\dfrac{1}{\sqrt{2}}$ can be rationalized by multiplication with $\dfrac{\sqrt{2}}{\sqrt{2}}$; the result is $\sqrt{2}/2$.

In general, if a radical appears as a multiplicative factor in the denominator, it can be eliminated by multiplying both numerator and denominator by the radical.

Example 7-14. Rationalize the fraction $\dfrac{3\sqrt{3}}{2\sqrt{5}}$. This is achieved by multiplying by $\dfrac{\sqrt{5}}{\sqrt{5}}$; the result is $\dfrac{3\sqrt{3}\sqrt{5}}{10} = \dfrac{3\sqrt{15}}{10}$.

Rationalizing the denominator usually makes the numerator more complicated. The main advantage of rationalization is that it permits the use of tables in the approximate numerical evaluation of expressions involving radicals. It is much easier to divide a multidigit number by the number with few digits than the other way around. For example, evaluating $\dfrac{1}{\sqrt{2}}$ by division in the approximate form $\dfrac{1}{1.414}$ is much more work than division in the rationalized form $\sqrt{2}/2 = \dfrac{1.414}{2}$, where the division to 0.707 is almost trivial.

Addition and subtraction of radicals. Addition and subtraction with radicals are limited to cases in which the radical portions are identical. For example, $2\sqrt[3]{2} + 3\sqrt[3]{2} = 5\sqrt[3]{2}$. However, $\sqrt{2} + \sqrt{3}$ cannot be substantially simplified.

Radical equations. Radicals occasionally appear in equations. They can be eliminated by raising the entire equation to appropriate powers. For example, in the simple equation $\sqrt{x} = 3$, the radical is eliminated by squaring both sides to yield $x = 9$. It should, however, be remembered that the equation resulting from raising an equation to a power may have more solutions than the original equation. It is therefore necessary to check all solutions in the original equation. For example, $\sqrt{x} = -2$ is an equation with no real solution for x, even though the squared equation $x = 4$ has a perfectly normal solution.

In the equation $4 = x - \sqrt{x}$ it is not sufficient to simply square both sides of the equation because the square root will persist; $16 = x^2 - 2x\sqrt{x} + x$. It is necessary to have the radical alone on one side of the equation as $\sqrt{x} = x - 4$ before taking the power. Now the result is the equation $x = x^2 - 8x + 16$.

Example 7-15. Eliminate the radical in the equation $x - \dfrac{1}{\sqrt{x}} = 1$.

The equation is first regrouped as $\dfrac{1}{\sqrt{x}} = x - 1$ and then squared:

$\dfrac{1}{x} = x^2 - 2x + 1$.

Tables of roots. Approximate decimal values of roots, particularly square roots, are available on many slide rules, electronic calculators, and high-speed computers, but there are also extensive published tables of square, cube, and higher-order roots. Most mathematical handbooks contain such tables. A small table of square and cube roots is presented in Appendix A. From that table, for example, $\sqrt{6}$ can be found to be 2.4495.

Example 7-16. Find $\sqrt[3]{2}$ from the tables in the appendix. This is given in row $n = 2$, column $\sqrt[3]{n}$. It is 1.2599.

EXPONENTIAL FUNCTIONS

If c is a constant and x is a variable, there are two common functional forms utilizing these as base and power. The form x^c is a *power function*; the graphic form and many of the functional properties have been described in Chapters 3 and 6. The other form (c^x) is known as the *exponential function*. In radiological applications, many of the relationships are exponential. These relationships include nuclear decay; x and γ beam attenuation; light transmittance through film; cell survival; charge and discharge of electrical capacitors; and light emission with time in phosphorescence.

ORIGIN AND SIGNIFICANCE. Consider the decay of 400,000 nuclei of ^{99m}Tc. In 6 hours, half of these will decay, leaving 200,000 nuclei. During the next 6 hours half of the remaining nuclei will decay, leaving 100,000 nuclei. After another 6 hours, only half of these, or 50,000, will be left, and so on. Each 6-hour period, or *half-life*, reduces the number of nuclei to half of the previous amount (Fig. 7-1).

As another example, consider the unrestricted growth of a cell population. Assume that, starting from a single cell, each cell will divide into two within 1 day. At the end of the first day, the single cell has become 2 cells. On the second day, the 2 cells become 4, and each day the number of cells doubles (Fig. 7-2).

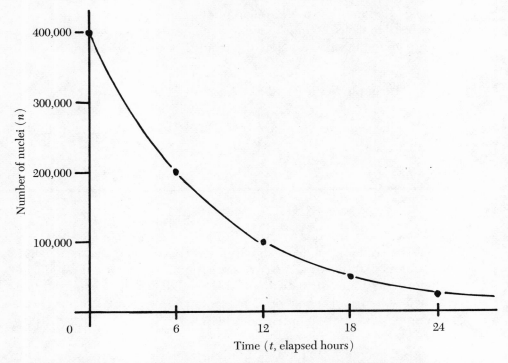

Fig. 7-1. The number of ^{99m}Tc nuclei present beginning with 400,000 nuclei as a function of time. The dots represent the numbers that are readily calculated from the 6 hour half-life; the smooth curve is the function $n = 2^{-t}$.

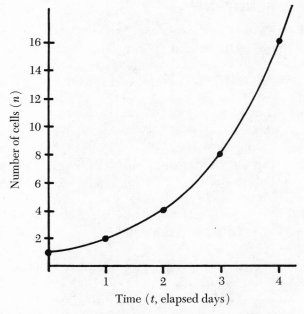

Fig. 7-2. The growth of an unrestricted cell population with a generation time of one day. The functional relationship indicated by the curve is the exponential $n = 2^t$.

These two examples represent exponential relationships. In both *the change in the amount is proportional to the original amount*. This property can be described in another way: For a given interval of the independent variable, regardless where the interval is taken, the fractional change in the dependent variable is the same. Using delta (Δ) to signify change, x for the independent, and y for the dependent variable, we can write this as follows:

$$\frac{\Delta y}{\Delta x} = cy$$

Formula 7-10

In this expression, c is a constant of proportionality. Since $\frac{\Delta y}{\Delta x}$ represents the slope, this formula gives a simple relationship between the slope and the dependent variable.

MATHEMATICAL PROPERTIES. The functional form of the exponential relationship can be written as follows:

$$y = Ka^{bx}$$

Formula 7-11

where K, a, and b are constants. As examples, the smooth line in Fig. 7-1 is $400,000 \, (2^{-1/6})$ ($K = 400,000$, $a = 2$, $b = -1/6$, and $x = t$). At $x = 0$, $a^{bx} = a^0 = 1$; thus at $x = 0$ the y of formula 7-11 is $y = K$, regardless of the values of a or b. In the fairly common case where $K = 1$, $y = 1$ at $x = 0$.

If b is positive, the function $y = Ka^{bx}$ is called a *positive exponential*. Fig. 7-2 is a typical example. A positive exponential starts at the y-axis with a nonzero value and gets farther and farther from the x-axis as the value of x increases; at any point, the slope is positive.

If b in formula 7-11 is negative, the function y is called a *negative exponential*. Fig. 7-1 is a typical example. Here the function starts with a nonzero value at the y-axis and approaches the x-axis ever more closely as x increases. Notice that neither the positive nor the negative function ever actually touches or crosses the x-axis. Almost all the exponential relationships of importance in radiology are of the negative exponential type.

As x becomes larger and larger, the positive exponential function becomes enormous. For example, consider the case shown in Fig. 7-2. Ten days after starting from a single cell, the population is at $1,024$ cells; at 20 days it is at 1.05×10^6 cells; at 30 days, there are 1.07×10^9 cells (roughly 1 gm for typical cells); and by 50 days, there are 1.13×10^{15} cells (about 1 metric ton).

As x becomes larger and larger with a negative exponential, the value of y gets closer and closer to zero until it can be effectively considered zero. For example, $2^{-10} \cong 1/1,000$ and $2^{-20} \cong 1.0 \times 10^{-6}$. This has important practical consequences; after a long enough time a radioactive material will have decayed to a point at which its activity is insignificant.

A common representation in radiology utilizes the convenient base $a = 2$. For nuclear decay the half-life (T) is the time required for a decay to half of the activity. From an initial activity (A_o) the activity (A) at any later time (t) is:

$$\boxed{A = A_o 2^{-t/T}}$$

Formula 7-12

Example 7-17. The half-life for ^{137}Cs is about 30 years. What is the activity of a 28 mCi source when it is 10 years old? The activity will be $28 \times 2^{-10/30} = 28 \times 2^{-1/3}$; $2^{-1/3}$ is $\frac{1}{\sqrt[3]{2}}$; $\sqrt[3]{2} \cong 1.2599$. Thus the activity is $^{28}/_{1.2599} \cong 22$ mCi.

Attenuation can be written in terms of the "half-value layers" (HVL). For an initial intensity, I_o, the intensity at any depth (x) will be:

$$I = I_o \, 2^{-x/_{HVL}}$$

Formula 7-13

provided that HVL does not change with depth.

Example 7-18. The HVL for ^{60}Co gamma rays in lead is about 1.2 cm. What would be the *transmission* (I/I_o) for ^{60}Co gamma rays in 6 cm of lead? Since we have 5 HVLs($^6/_{1.2}$), the transmission will be $2^{-5} = {}^1/_{32} \cong 0.03$, or 3%.

Another common base is 10. Attenuation can be described in terms of tenth-value layers (TVLs). In the next chapter, the relationship between TVLs and HVLs will be explored. A base 10 is also used in describing the light absorption of a developed film. The transmission (T) of light through a film is:

$$T = 10^{-D}$$

Formula 7-14

where D is known as the *density*.

Example 7-19. What percent of incident light is transmitted by a film of a density equal to 1? $T = 10^{-1} = {}^1/_{10}$, or 10%.

Base of the natural numbers. The most common base for exponential functions is the value e, which is approximately 2.718. It is variously known as the *base of the natural numbers*, "Euler's constant," or "Euler's number."*

Two features of e may indicate why it is such a popular base for exponential functions. When graphed, the functions $y = e^x$ and $y = e^{-x}$ have a slope equal to $+1$ and -1, respectively, at the y-axis. (For the base 2, a slope of $+1$ corresponds to the function $y = 2^{0.693x}$). A second advantage of e as a base is the approximation of $y = e^x$ or $y = e^{-x}$ when x is small. Then, $e^x \cong 1 + x$ and $e^{-x} \cong 1 - x$, provided $x \ll 1$.

---

*Whereas it is true that e is taken from Euler's name, it must not be confused with another constant also ascribed to Euler.

Example 7-20. What is the slope at the y-axis of the exponential function $y = e^{2x}$? For values of x that are small (near the y-axis) $e^{2x} \cong 1 + 2x$. $1 + 2x$ is a straight line with slope 2.

The function $y = e^x$ is sometimes known as the *exponential function* and is often written as $e^x = \exp(x)$.

Many important exponential formulas in radiology use the base e. For example, attenuation can be written as follows:

$$I = I_o e^{-\mu x} \qquad \text{Formula 7-15}$$

Here I and I_o are defined as in formula 7-13, and μ is the *attenuation coefficient*, that is, the fraction of the incident photons removed from a beam per unit of thickness of material.

Exponential approach. When a radioactive nucleus decays, one or more daughter nuclei are created. If these are stable, a sample containing a large number of the radioactive parent nuclei will contain an increasing number of daughter nuclei as time passes. An example of this situation is shown in Fig. 7-3 for the decay of ^{60}Co in $5\frac{1}{4}$ years. With a pure sample of ^{60}Co, there is no ^{60}Ni present originally, but after $5\frac{1}{4}$ years, half the ^{60}Co has changed to ^{60}Ni. After $10\frac{1}{2}$ years, only one fourth of the original ^{60}Co nuclei remains unchanged; three-fourths of the nuclei have changed to ^{60}Ni. As time increases,

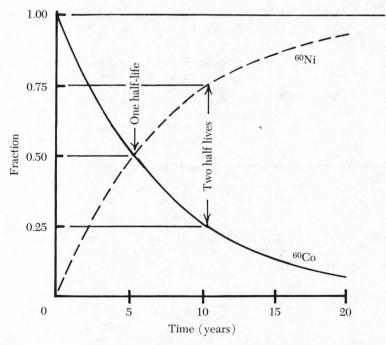

Fig. 7-3. The decay of a pure sample of ^{60}Co into ^{60}Ni. The decay of each ^{60}Co nucleus results in the creation of a ^{60}Ni nucleus.

the number of ^{60}Ni nuclei will approach the initial number of ^{60}Co nuclei. For this example, the number of cobalt nuclei (N^c) as a function of time is described by the radioactive decay equivalent of formula 7-15:

$$N^c = N_o^c e^{-\lambda t} \qquad \text{Formula 7-16}$$

N_o^c is the initial number of cobalt nuclei, and λ is the *decay constant* for cobalt—the probability of decay of a nucleus per unit of time. The number of cobalt nuclei decayed (N) is the initial less the present number:

$$N = N_o^c - N^c = N_o^c - N_o^c e^{-\lambda t} = N_o^c (1 - e^{-\lambda t}) \qquad \text{Formula 7-17}$$

Because all the ^{60}Co decays to ^{60}Ni, N is also the number of nickel nuclei.

The growth of ^{60}Ni in this example is a typical case of *exponential approach*. There are other examples in radiology, such as the production of stable nuclides through nuclear reactions or through the decay of radioactive parents.

Although the exponential approach formulas are usually written with e as the base, other bases may be used. For example, formula 7-17 can be written in terms of the half-life (T) as follows:

$$N = N_o(1 - 2^{-t/T}) \qquad \text{Formula 7-18}$$

Example 7-21. For a temporary implant with short–half-life radionuclides, the dose delivered is proportional to the "activity lost" (A_L). This value is simply the initial activity (A_o) less the activity removed (A) at the end of the implant. Express this in terms of the half-life. The activity obeys formula 7-12, that is, $A = A_o 2^{-t/T}$. Thus the activity lost will be $A_L = A_o (1 - 2^{-t/T})$.

Example 7-22. Use the result of example 7-21 to find the activity lost during a 5.4-day implant of 50 mCi of ^{198}Au (half-life 2.7 days). Here, $A_o = 50$, $t = 5.4$, $T = 2.7$, and $t/T = 2$; thus $A_L = 50 (1 - 2^{-2}) = 50(1 - 1/4) = 50(3/4) = 37.5$ mCi.

CHAPTER REVIEW

1. What is the law of exponents for multiplication and division?
2. What is the law of exponents for the power of a power?
3. What is the significance of the zero power?
4. What is the numerical value of the zero power?
5. What is the significance of a negative power?
6. What does a fractional power represent?
7. What is a radical?
8. What conditions must be met to reduce a radical to a lower order?
9. How are radical equations handled?
10. What condition must be met for dependence to be exponential?
11. In the exponential relationship, is the variable in the base or the power?
12. For large values of the independent

variable, what values will a positive exponential have?

13. What value does a negative exponential approach as the independent variable becomes large?
14. What numbers make a suitable base for exponential functions?
15. What is "e"?
16. What is meant by "exponential approach"?

PROBLEMS

Problems paralleling chapter examples

1. **(7-1)** Simplify $(a^5b^2)(ab^3c^2)$.
2. **(7-2)** Simplify $\dfrac{w^4v^2}{w^2v}$.
3. **(7-3)** Simplify $\dfrac{5.0 \times 10^4}{2.5 \times 10^2}$.
4. **(7-4)** Simplify $(5^2)^3$.
5. **(7-6)** Express $\left[\dfrac{x^5}{y}\right]^2 \quad \left[\dfrac{1}{xy}\right]^3$ without parentheses.
6. **(7-7)** What is the value of 10^0?
7. **(7-8)** Eliminate the denominator in the expression $\dfrac{x^2}{y^2}$.
8. **(7-9)** What is the value of $16^{1/4}$?
9. **(7-10)** What is the value of $8^{2/3}$?
10. **(7-11)** Express the ninth root of 64 as a cube root.
11. **(7-12)** Express $3\sqrt[3]{4}$ as a single number entirely within the radical sign.
12. **(7-13)** Simplify $\sqrt{9/32}$.
13. **(7-14)** Rationalize $\dfrac{2}{\sqrt{7}}$.
14. **(7-15)** Eliminate the radical in the equation $1 - \sqrt{x} = x + 2\sqrt{x}$.
15. **(7-16)** Find $\sqrt{7}$ using the tables in Appendix A.
16. **(7-17)** The half-life of ^{99m}Tc is 6 hours. What is the activity of 10 mCi after 3 hours?
17. **(7-18)** At high attenuation the HVL in lead for 100 kVp x-rays is about 0.24 mm. "Two-pound lead" (2 lb/feet²) is approximately $\frac{1}{32}$ inch thick, or 0.79 mm. Approximately how many HVL is this for 100 kVp?
18. **(7-19)** What percent of light is transmitted through a film of density 2?
19. **(7-20)** What is the slope of the function e^{-3r} near the y-axis?

20. **(7-21)** The intensity (I) of light transmitted through a film of density (D) can be related to the incident intensity (I_o) as $I = I_o\, 10^{-D}$ by employing formula 7-14. What is the "intensity lost" in such a film?

Problems related to this chapter

21. Express as a number without exponent:
    a. 3^3
    b. $4^{1/2}$
    c. 5^2
    d. 2^{10}
    e. 4^5
    f. $8^{2/3}$
22. Simplify:
    a. $(x^{1/2})^2$
    b. $(x^2)^{1/2}$
    c. x^3x^{-4}
    d. $\dfrac{x^7}{x^{-3}}$
    e. $\dfrac{x^{15}}{x^{14}}$
23. Find an approximate (three-figure) numerical value for:
    a. e^0
    b. e^1
    c. e^{-1}
    d. e^{-2}
    e. e^{+2}
24. Find an approximate (three-figure) numerical value for (express as a decimal number):
    a. $10^{0.5}$
    b. 10^{-1}
    c. $\dfrac{1}{\sqrt{10}}$
    d. 2^{-1}
    e. 2^{-5}
25. Rationalize (that is, eliminate the square root sign in the denominator):
    a. $\dfrac{1}{\sqrt{2}}$
    b. $\dfrac{3}{\sqrt{5}}$
26. Calculate the following:
    a. 2^3
    b. $(-3)^2$
    c. $4^{1/2}$
    d. $\sqrt[3]{27}$
    e. $16^{3/2}$

27. If $y = x^2$, write the following expressions in terms of x (for example, $y^2 = x^4$):
    a. $\sqrt{y}$ c. $y^{1/2}$
    b. y^3 d. y^0
28. Simplify the following (for example, $\dfrac{x^3}{x}$ $= x^2$):
    a. $\dfrac{x^5(x^{-2})}{x^4}$ b. $\dfrac{(x^3 - x^5)}{x^4(1 + x^2)}$
29. If $e^{2.3} \cong 10$, then what is $e^{4.6}$?
30. Give the values for e^{-x} (for example, for $x = 1$, $e^{-x} \cong 0.37$):
    a. when $x = 0$
    b. when x gets very large

Objective questions

31. The product $2^1 \times 2^3$ is equal to:
    a. $1^2 \times 3^2$ d. 4^4
    b. 2^4 e. 4^3
    c. 2^3
32. The value of 6^0 is:
    a. 0   d. 6
    b. $\frac{1}{6}$ e. 36
    c. 1
33. Identify the curve of the function $y = Ae^{-bx}$ in Fig. 7-4 by its letter label.

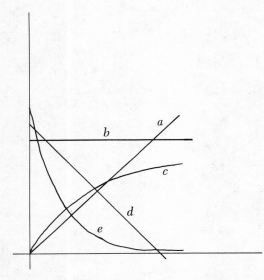

Fig. 7-4. Graphs of various functions.

34. The statement "y is inversely related to the square of x" can be written as:
    a. $x = y^2$ d. $y = \dfrac{1}{x^2}$
    b. $y = x^2$
    c. $x = \dfrac{1}{y^2}$

35. The power relationship shown in Fig. 7-5 is:
    a. linear
    b. square (or quadratic)
    c. inverse (or hyperbolic)
    d. inverse square

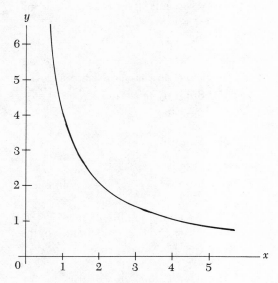

Fig. 7-5. A power relationship.

36. The fraction $\dfrac{1}{\sqrt{2}}$ is equal to
    a. $\frac{1}{4}$ d. $\frac{1}{2}$
    b. $\sqrt{2}$ e. $\dfrac{\sqrt{2}}{4}$
    c. $2^{-1/2}$
37. A simplified version of $\sqrt{216}$ is:
    a. $6\sqrt{6}$
    b. $5\sqrt{5}$
    c. $4\sqrt{4}$
    d. $3\sqrt{3}$
    e. $2\sqrt{2}$
38. As a decimal, 2^{-2} is equal to:
    a. 0.0   d. 1.0
    b. 0.25   e. −4.0
    c. 0.5
39. The solution to the equation $\sqrt[3]{x} = 8$ is:
    a. $x = 2$
    b. $x = 16$
    c. $x = 24$
    d. $x = 128$
    e. $x = 512$

40. In some situations the number of cells killed (the change in the number of cells) is proportional to the product of the initial number of cells and the dose. This relationship is:
    a. quadratic
    b. linear
    c. inverse square
    d. negative exponential
    e. positive exponential

41. The output of most x-ray units changes as the inverse square of the distance. Increasing the distance a factor of 10 will change the output by a factor of:
    a. $\sqrt{10}$ d. 1
    b. 100   e. $1/100$
    c. 10

CHAPTER 8

Logarithms

Before the advent of the inexpensive electronic calculator, logarithms had a major function in the evaluation of products, quotients, or roots. Now they still perform several important functions. For example, logarithms can be used to eliminate exponents in an algebraic expression, to express very large numbers in a more convenient form, and to compress the scale on graphs that extend over several orders of magnitude.

POWERS OF TEN—COMMON LOGARITHMS

In Chapter 2 on scientific notation we saw that it is frequently convenient to express numbers in two parts. The first part is a number of moderate size and the second part is a *power of ten*. Particularly if we are just interested in an approximation, the "order of magnitude" of a quantity, the power of ten may be all we want to know.

The power of ten is an exponential expression with ten as the base. For very large and very small numbers it is particularly convenient to use the power of ten formulation. With this notation, a ten-digit calculator can display numbers from 10^{-99} to 10^{99} with a six-figure accuracy. Without the use of powers of ten, this range of values would require a display of over 105 digits.

The power of ten of a number is called the *characteristic* of this number in the notation of the *common logarithms*. For example, the characteristic for the number 15 (1.5×10^1) is 1; for 100 (10^2) it is 2; for 0.045 (4.5×10^{-2}) it is -2. For numbers that are exact powers of ten, the entire logarithm is the characteristic. That is:

$$\log(10^n) = n \qquad \text{Formula 8-1}$$

Here, "log" is read as "the common logarithm of."

> **Example 8-1.** What is the common logarithm of 0.01? Since 0.01 is equal to 10^{-2}, $\log 0.01 = -2$.

Thus:

$$\text{If } \log(x) = a, \text{ then } x = 10^a \qquad \text{Formula 8-2}$$

What about numbers that are not exact powers of 10? Consider 37; this number is between 10, whose logarithm is 1.0, and 100, whose logarithm is 2.0. Thus we expect the logarithm of 37 to have a value between 1.0 and 2.0.

THE MANTISSA. When we have a number in scientific notation, for example, 4.2×10^5, the power of ten, 5 in this case, is readily converted into the characteristic of the logarithm of the number, in our case log (4.2) + 5. There remains a number between 1 and 10, here 4.2, whose logarithm is between 0 (the log of 1) and 1 (the log of 10). The logarithm of this number is the *mantissa*; it is always represented as a decimal. Numbers that differ from one another only in powers of ten will all have the same mantissa but different characteristics. *The common logarithm is the sum of the mantissa and the characteristic.*

The numerical value of the mantissa is chosen in accordance with formula 8-2. For example, a mantissa of 0.5 would be the logarithm of $10^{0.5} = 10^{1/2} = \sqrt{10} \cong 3.16$; that is, the log (3.16) $\cong$ 0.5.

> **Example 8-2.** Use $3.16 = 10^{0.5}$ to find the common logarithm of 31.6. In scientific notation, $31.6 = 3.16 \times 10^1$. For this, the mantissa is 0.5 and the characteristic is 1. Thus the common logarithm is log(31.6) = 1.5.

For the evaluation of most mantissas, we will rely on published tables or electronic calculation. A table of logarithms is presented in Appendix A; more extensive tables can be found in standard mathematical handbooks.

FINDING THE LOGARITHM. To find the logarithm of a number x, we first write x in scientific notation:

$$x = a \times 10^b$$

where $1 \le a < 10$ and b is an integer. The logarithm of x, $\log(x)$, will have a characteristic b and a mantissa equal to $\log(a)$:

$$\boxed{\log(a \times 10^b) = b + \log(a)}$$ **Formula 8-3**

For the following examples, $\log(a)$ can be found in the tables in the Appendix.

> **Example 8-3.** Find log(27). The scientific notation for this is 2.7×10^1. The characteristic is 1; the mantissa is found to be 0.431. Thus log(27) = 1.431.

> **Example 8-4.** Find log(0.0041). The scientific notation for this is 4.1×10^{-3}. The characteristic is -3, and the mantissa is 0.613. Thus log (0.0041) = $-3 + 0.613 = -2.387$.

In cases where the characteristic is negative, it was customary to maintain a positive mantissa and a negative characteristic by one of several techniques.

(For example, the log of 0.05 has a characteristic of -2 and a mantissa of 0.699. This could be written as $\bar{2}.699$, in which the bar over the 2 indicates a negative value. It is sometimes written as $-10 + 8.699$.) Since the advent of electronic calculation, however, this is an obsolete practice.

Formal definition and log of the inverse. Formula 8-2 can be rewritten as a definition of the common logarithm as follows:

$$x = 10^{\log(x)}$$

Formula 8-4

This shows that *the common logarithm is the power to which 10 is raised to give the desired quantity.* This is obviously consistent with formula 8-1.

As there is no (real) power to which ten can be raised to yield a negative result, there are no logarithms of negative numbers.

The logarithm of an inverse quantity $1/x$ follows directly from formula 8-4. The inverse of this formula is as follows:

$$1/x = \frac{1}{10^{\log(x)}}$$

A power in the denominator can be moved to the numerator by changing the sign of the power: $\dfrac{1}{x} = 10^{\log(1/x)} = 10^{-\log(x)}$, but comparing these two forms we see:

$$\log(1/x) = -\log(x)$$

Formula 8-5

Example 8-5. What is $\log(\frac{1}{2})$? This is $-\log(2)$; and $\log(2) = 0.301$. Thus, $\log(\frac{1}{2}) = -0.301$.

ANTILOGARITHMS

In the preceding section we saw that if $\log(x) = y$ and we are given x, we can find y. The reverse process, finding x when y is given, is known as *taking the antilog*. This can be written as $x = \text{antilog}(y)$, or, more commonly, as the exponential expression $x = 10^y$.

The defining formula for logarithms (formula 8-4):

$$x = 10^{\log(x)}$$

shows one way to find a number whose logarithm is known. Written in terms of the antilog of y, where $y = \log(x)$ and $\text{antilog}(y) = x$, this formula is:

$$\text{antilog}(y) = 10^y$$

Formula 8-6

This formula can sometimes be used to evaluate antilogarithms. If an electronic calculator has 10^x available as a standard function, the use is obvious.

Probably the most common method for finding antilogs is based on the logarithm tables. This method reverses the technique for finding logarithms. The position of the mantissa is found in the table and the row and/or column of the position in the table determines the antilog. For example, the antilog of 0.74 is found in the tables for the value of $x = 5.5$ (see Appendix A).

> **Example 8-6.** Find the antilog of 0.85. This is located in row 7 and column 0.1. Thus the antilog(0.85) is 7.1.

For those cases in which the characteristic is not zero, it is handled separately; it converts directly to the power of ten in scientific notation. For example, antilog 4.475 = [antilog(0.475)] $\times$ 10^4 = 3.0 $\times$ 10^4.

> **Example 8-7.** Find the antilog of 7.820. This has a characteristic of 7. The antilog of the mantissa is 6.6. Thus the antilog(7.820) = 6.6 $\times$ 10^7.

BASIC PRINCIPLES OF LOGARITHMS

The mathematical properties of logarithms follow from the defining formula (formula 8-4) and the properties of exponents.

MULTIPLICATION AND DIVISION. Formula 8-4 can be written for x and y as $x = 10^{\log(x)}$ and $y = 10^{\log(y)}$. If these are multiplied, then

$$xy = 10^{\log(x)}10^{\log(y)}$$

The expression on the right can be handled by formula 7-1 for exponents so that:

$$xy = 10^{\log(x)}10^{\log(y)} = 10^{\log(x)+\log(y)}$$

However, the product xy itself must obey formula 8-4:

$$xy = 10^{\log(xy)}$$

Equating these two expressions produces the interesting relationship:

$$\boxed{\log(xy) = \log(x) + \log(y)} \qquad \text{Formula 8-7}$$

This formula is extremely important. It reduces a product to an addition; addition is relatively easy to carry out. This relationship was the basis for the design of the slide rule; it is now used electronically for multiplication in some calculations.

> **Example 8-8.** Verify formula 8-7 for the case of $x = 2, y = 5$. In this case $xy = 10$; the logarithms are $\log(10) = 1$, $\log 2 = 0.301$, and $\log 5 = 0.699$. Since $0.301 + 0.699 = 1.0$, formula 8-7 is satisfied.

> **Example 8-9.** Derive a formula for $\log(x^3)$ in terms of $\log(x)$. The expression x^3 can be written as x^2x; thus $\log(x^3) = \log(x^2x) = \log(x^2)$

$+ \log(x)$. $\text{Log}(x^2) = \log(x) + \log(x)$.   Thus $\log(x^3) = \log(x) + \log(x) + \log(x) = 3 \log(x)$.

The division formula is derived in a manner analogous to that for formula 8-7.

$$\frac{x}{y} = \frac{10^{\log(x)}}{10^{\log(y)}} = 10^{\log(x)}10^{-\log(y)} = 10^{\log(x)-\log(y)} = 10^{\log(x/y)}$$

or

$$\log(x/y) = \log(x) - \log(y) \qquad \text{Formula 8-8}$$

This formula can also be derived by considering division as the multiplication of the inverse.

Example 8-10. Express the equation $\log N = \log(N_0) - \dfrac{d}{D_0}$ in terms of a single logarithm. Subtracting $\log(N_0)$ from both sides results in the equation $\log(N) - \log(N_0) = -\dfrac{d}{D_0}$; the two logarithms can be combined according to formula 8-8 to give $\log\left(\dfrac{N}{N_0}\right) = -\dfrac{d}{D_0}$.

Example 8-11. Eliminate the minus sign in the result of example 8-10. Both sides can be multiplied by -1 to yield $-\log\left(\dfrac{N}{N_0}\right) = \dfrac{d}{D_0}$. Formula 8-5 shows that the minus sign in front of a logarithm can be eliminated by using the logarithm of the inverse: $\log\left(\dfrac{N_0}{N}\right) = \dfrac{d}{D_0}$.

The logarithm of powers. Example 8-9 illustrates a formula that is readily derived from formula 8-7 for integral powers:

$$\boxed{\log x^n = n \log x} \qquad \text{Formula 8-9}$$

Note that formula 8-1 is a special case of formula 8-9 with $x = 10$. Also, formula 8-5 is a special case with $n = -1$.

This formula will be derived for any power (k) by considering the k-th power of the defining formula for logarithms (formula 8-4):

$$x^k = 10^{\log x^k}$$

But formula 7-3 for the power of a power can be used to show the following:

$$x^k = [10^{\log(x)}]^k = 10^{(k)\log(x)}$$

This shows that formula 8-9 applies to all powers and not just integer powers.

Example 8-12. The half-value layer (HVL) for a ^{60}Co beam is about 1.2 cm of lead; 2.0 cm would be about $1^2/_3$ or $5/_3$ HVL. The transmission (T) through 2 cm of lead is $T = 2^{-5/_3}$. Find the logarithm of this quantity, and by taking its antilogarithm, find the transmission. $\text{Log}(T) = \log(2^{-5/_3}) = -5/_3 \log 2 \cong -5/_3(0.301) = -0.502$. T is the antilog of this quantity. This negative log can be solved either by noting that it refers to an inverse or by changing it to $-1 + 0.498$; we will use the latter form here and evaluate as antilog$(0.498) \times 10^{-1} \cong 3.1 \times 10^{-1} = 0.31$.

The process used in example 8-12, that is, taking the logarithm, multiplying by the power, and taking the antilogarithm, is the way in which virtually all fractional powers are evaluated. Fractional powers are very common; in radiological applications the exponential relationships are the most frequent sources.

APPLICATIONS TO ALGEBRA. The logarithm is the mechanism used to formally eliminate a power by means of formula 8-9. Consider the equation for nuclear decay: $N = N_0 e^{-\lambda t}$; here N is the number of nuclei present at time t, N_0 is the initial number, λ is the decay constant, and e is the base of the natural numbers. Suppose we wish to "solve" for t. Our usual methods of solution given in Chapter 3 will not be adequate, since t appears in a power. However, if we take the logarithm of both sides of this equation we find the following:

$$\log(N) = \log(N_0 e^{-\lambda t}) = \log(N_0) + \log(e^{-\lambda t}) = \log(N_0) - (\lambda t) \log(e)$$

With this change the equation can be solved for t as follows:

$$t = \frac{\log\left(\dfrac{N_0}{N}\right)}{\lambda \log(e)}$$

Example 8-13. The transmission of light (T) through a film of density D is $T = 10^{-D}$. Solve this equation for D. Here we take the logarithm to obtain $\log(T) = -(D) \log 10$. Since $\log 10 = 1$, $\log(T) = -D$, or $D = -\log(T)$, or $\log(1/_T)$.

In addition to actual solution of equations containing powers, logarithms offer a method for expressing exponential relationships. Consider the following two equations:

$$y = a^x$$

and

$$\log (y) = x \log a$$

The first of these two equations can be said to be in *exponential form*, and the second is in the *logarithmic form*. These two equations are equivalent ways to express the relationship between the variables x and y. The choice between the forms for actual use is a matter of convenience.

OTHER LOGARITHMS

The logarithms discussed up to this point are called common logarithms. In some instances, other forms are preferable.

LOGARITHMS OF VARIOUS BASES. The logarithm is a power to which a suitable base is raised to result in a certain quantity. Formula 8-4, the basic definition of the common logarithm, can be generalized to the following form:

$$x = a^{\log_a(x)}$$

Formula 8-10

The new entity $\log_a(x)$ is read as "the logarithm of x to the base a." Common logarithms have the base 10 (the subscript is usually omitted). In principle, any positive number except 1 is a possible base for logarithms. In practice, 10 and e are the most common bases; 2 is less common, but is becoming more important in the relatively new field of binary mathematics. Other bases are restricted almost entirely to mathematical formulas.

If we take the common logarithm of formula 8-10, we obtain:

$$\log(x) = \log[a^{\log_a(x)}] = \log_a(x)\,\log(a)$$

When this is solved for $\log_a(x)$, the result is:

$$\log_a(x) = \frac{\log(x)}{\log(a)}$$

Formula 8-11

This shows that the logarithm of a number to any base can be found readily from common logarithms.

Example 8-14. What is $\log_2(5)$? Formula 8-11 shows that $\log_2(5) = \dfrac{\log(5)}{\log(2)} = \dfrac{0.699}{0.301} = 2.32$.

Logarithms to bases other than 10 share many of the properties of common logarithms. All the formulas in this chapter that do not contain one or more numerical values apply to logarithms of any base. These formulas are 8-5, 8-7, 8-8, and 8-9. A drawback of all bases other than 10 is that they do not permit us to break a number into characteristic and mantissa. This makes actual computation with them a cumbersome procedure. One feature all bases share is that one is the logarithm of the base:

$$\log_a(a) = 1$$

Formula 8-12

This is frequently useful. For example, the equation $\dfrac{N}{N_0} = 2^{-t/T}$ is equal to $\log_2\left(\dfrac{N}{N_0}\right) = -t/T$; if any base other than 2 were used, logarithms would appear on both sides of the equal sign.

NATURAL LOGARITHMS. The most frequently used base other than 10 is the base of the natural numbers, $e \cong 2.72$, which appears in many exponential functions. The logarithms to the base e are usually called the *natural logarithms*, and e is sometimes called *the base of the natural logarithms*. The common logarithms are usually designated by "log" and the natural logarithms by "ln."

The relationship between natural logarithms and common logarithms is as follows:

$$\ln(x) \cong 2.30 \log(x) \qquad \text{Formula 8-13}$$

Because natural logarithms appear so frequently, they are often tabulated. The term "antilogarithms" is never used in conjunction with natural logarithms; the inverse of a natural logarithm is always represented in the exponential form (e^x).

Example 8-15. Find $\ln(2)$. The tables in Appendix A give $\log(2) = 0.301$. Thus $\ln(2) \cong 2.30(0.301) = 0.692$ (a more exact calculation gives 0.693).

Example 8-16. The intensity (I) of a monoenergetic photon beam of initial intensity I_0 in a uniform absorber can be expressed as $I = I_0 e^{-\mu x}$ where μ is the linear attenuation coefficient and x is the thickness of the material. Use natural logarithms to express this in a logarithmic form using only one logarithm. The logarithm of this expression is $\ln I = \ln I_0 - \mu x \, (\ln e)$. According to formula 8-12, $\ln e = 1$. Then $\ln I = \ln I_0 - \mu x$, $\ln I - \ln I_0 = -\mu x$, or $\ln\left(\dfrac{I_0}{I}\right) = \mu x$.

In the previous chapter it was noted that exponential relationships can be expressed in several ways. For example, radioactive decay can be expressed as $\dfrac{N}{N_0} = e^{-\lambda t} = 2^{-t/T}$, where N_0 is the initial number of nuclei, N is the number at time t, λ is the decay constant, and T is the half-life. There is a relationship between the half-life and the decay constant; this relationship is found by taking the natural logarithm of the equation $e^{-\lambda t} = 2^{-t/T}$. This yields $-\lambda t = -(t/T) \ln 2$; canceling t and multiplying by -1 gives $\lambda = \dfrac{\ln 2}{T} = \dfrac{0.693}{T}$. A similar relationship exists between the half-value layer and the attenuation coefficient.

LOGARITHMS IN GRAPHS

LOGARITHMIC FUNCTIONS. The function $y = \log(x)$ is plotted in Fig. 8-1. This is just the exponential function discussed in Chapter 7 reflected about the y-axis and rotated clockwise 90 degrees. The logarithmic relationship can be expressed in terms of the exponential relationship; it is traditional to use the

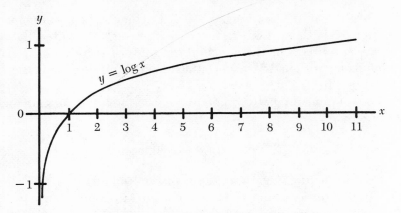

Fig. 8-1. The graph of the function $y = \log (x)$.

exponential rather than the logarithmic form for graphic purposes. Thus the graph of the logarithmic function is relatively rare.

The general features of the logarithmic function are readily seen in Fig. 8-1. The x intercept is $x = 1 (10^0 = 1)$. There is no y intercept and no negative values of x. For large values of x, the logarithmic function increases slowly as x increases; however, there is no upper limit to the value of $\ln(x)$ as x gets larger and larger. As x gets smaller and smaller, $\ln(x)$ decreases; as x approaches zero, $\log(x)$ approaches negative infinity.

Log scales. Logarithmic scales are extremely important in graphing. For instance, they permit the compression of a scale in such a way that variations over several orders of magnitude can be visualized. Fig. 8-2 shows a graph of the function $y = e^{-x^2}$ and the logarithm of the same function. For values $x \geq 2$ the function e^{-x^2} is so small that the graph of the function is essentially on top of the x-axis. From the graph of e^{-x^2} alone it would be impossible to say, for example, whether or not the function is exactly zero at, say $x = 3$, or if it is decreasing at $x = 2.5$. On the other hand, the graph of the logarithm of e^{-x^2} can be interpreted readily for these points. At least up to $x = 3$, the logarithm is negative and has a negative slope. The negative slope indicates that the function e^{-x^2} continues to decrease. The fact that the logarithm of e^{-x^2} does not drop all the way to negative infinity indicates that e^{-x^2} has no intercept in this range. Thus we see that the logarithm of a function may be a more suitable item to graph than the function itself.

It is possible to evaluate the logarithm of a function and then plot the result on Cartesian graph paper. But it is simpler and quicker to use graph paper on which one or both of the scales are logarithmic. An example of the vertical (y) axis being logarithmic is shown in Fig. 8-3. This is known as a *semilogarithmic* graph, since only one of the axes is logarithmic.

Along a logarithmic axis a change of a factor of 10 has a fixed distance regardless of the absolute amount. In fact, a change by any given factor is the same at all points on the scale. This scale does not have a point corresponding to zero. The relationship shown in Fig. 8-3 is the exponential relationship for

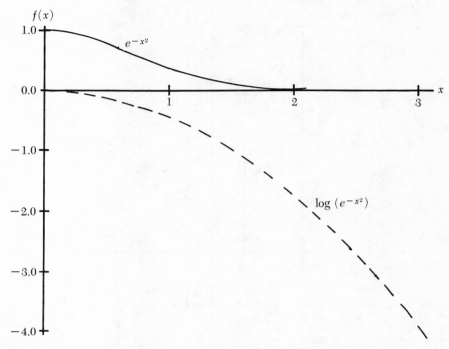

Fig. 8-2. The graph of e^{-x^2} and its logarithm.

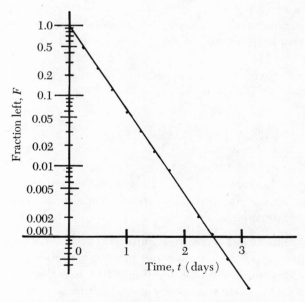

Fig. 8-3. The decay of ^{99m}Tc plotted on semilog graph paper. The fraction *(F)* left after a certain time *(t)* is $F = e^{-\lambda t}$.

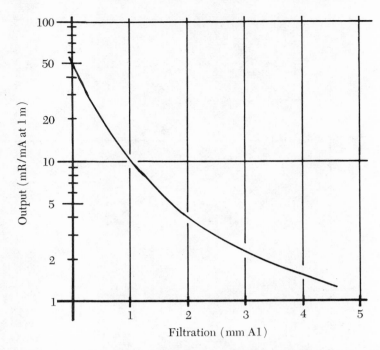

Fig. 8-4. The output of a certain x-ray tube as a function of added aluminum filtration.

the remaining fraction of ^{99m}Tc, $F = e^{-\lambda t}$. It can be seen that this exponential relationship appears as a straight line when plotted on semilogarithmic paper. This is a general feature of all true exponential relationships. The converse is also true: a function that appears as a straight line on semilogarithmic paper is exponential.

The exponential relationships can be explored algebraically. Consider the ^{99m}Tc example illustrated in Fig. 8-3. Written in terms of an exponential to base 2:

$F = 2^{-t/6}$, where t is expressed in hours. If we call the logarithm of F y:

$$y = \log(F) = {}^{-t}/_6 \log(2)$$

or

$$y = -\left[\frac{\log(2)}{6}\right] t \cong -\frac{0.301}{6} t \cong -0.050\, t$$

This is a linear relationship between y (or $\log F$) and t. Conversely, a linear relationship between the logarithm of the dependent variable and the independent variable is equivalent to an exponential relationship between the variables themselves.

> **Example 8-17.** Fig. 8-4 shows a typical relationship between the output (exposure) of an x-ray tube and the amount of added aluminum filtration. The plot is semilogarithmic. Is there an exponential relationship between the output and the thickness of aluminum? The graph is not a straight line on semilogarithmic paper. Thus the relationship is not exponential.

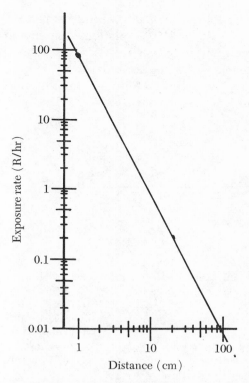

Fig. 8-5. The exposure rate from a 10 mg radium source. This graph has log-log scales.

In the case of a semilogarithmic graph of an exponential function, such as that shown in Fig. 8-3, the slope of the graph is proportional to the constant in the power. Also, a negative exponential will have a straight line with negative slope in a semilogarithmic plot, whereas a positive exponential will have a straight line with a positive slope.

Sometimes it is convenient to use logarithmic scales on both axes, known as a log-log plot; the graph paper is called *log-log paper*. The reasons for using log-log paper are similar to those for using semilogarithmic paper: either it is a convenient range for the scales or certain functional relationships will graph as straight lines on a log-log plot.

The functions that plot as straight lines in log-log graphs are power functions with both positive and negative (inverse) powers. An example of the exposure rate associated with a 10 mCi point source of radium is shown in Fig. 8-5. If the horizontal and vertical scales are equal, that is, if the width of a "cycle" or power of 10 is the same, the slope of the line is equal to the power of the functional relationship. For example, the relationship between the exposure rate and the distance from a point source is an inverse square; thus the slope of the line in Fig. 8-5 is −2.

Example 8-18. The exposure at a point behind a thick phantom is plotted as a function of kilovolt peak (kVp) for fixed millamperage on log-log paper. The result is a line that is approximately straight with a slope of +4.5. Write the relationship between the exposure X and kVp; assume that the output at kVp_0 is X_0. Since the line in a log-log plot is approximately straight, the relationship can be represented as a power. The slope of the line is +4.5; therefore the power is 4.5, or the output X is proportional to $kVp^{4.5}$. However, $X = X_0$ at $kVp = kVp_0$, or

$$X = X_0 \left(\frac{kVp}{kVp_0} \right)^{4.5}.$$

CHAPTER REVIEW

1. How are scientific notation and the characteristic of logarithms related? How are characteristics of logarithms obtained? What is the mantissa?
2. How are mantissas obtained in practical cases?
3. How is a number translated into its logarithm?
4. What is an antilogarithm?
5. What function is an antilog equivalent to?
6. How do the logarithms of a product relate to the logarithms of the separate factors?
7. How do the logarithms of a number and its inverse relate?
8. How are fractional powers evaluated?
9. Why is there no logarithm of zero?
10. What functional relationship is equivalent to the logarithmic relationship?
11. What are natural logarithms?
12. What is the relationship between common logarithms and natural logarithms?
13. What function(s) appear(s) as straight line(s) in a semilogarithmic graph?
14. How does the slope of a straight line in a log-log plot relate to the functional form of the variables?

PROBLEMS
Problems paralleling chapter examples

1. (8-1) What is the common logarithm of 1,000?
2. (8-2) $10^{0.25} = 1.78$. Use this to evaluate the common logarithm of 178.

3. (8-3) Find log(44).
4. (8-4) Find log(0.059).
5. (8-5) Find log $1/3$.
6. (8-6) Find the antilog of 0.36.
7. (8-7) Find the antilog of 4.91.
8. (8-9) Use formula 8-7 to derive an expression for log (x^4).
9. (8-11) Eliminate the negative sign in the formula $\log \dfrac{I}{I_0} = \frac{-x}{T}$.
10. (8-12) The half-life of ^{99m}Tc is 6 hours. Eight hours is $1\frac{1}{3} = \frac{4}{3}$ half-life. The fraction of ^{99m}Tc remaining after 8 hours is thus $2^{-4/3}$. Evaluate this using common logarithms.
11. (8-13) With uncontrolled cell doubling with a doubling time T, the number of cells present at any time (t) is $N = N_0\, 2^{t/T}$ where N_0 is the initial number of cells. Solve this equation for t.
12. (8-14) Find $\log_5(9)$.
13. (8-15) Find $\ln(3)$.
14. (8-16) Radioactive decay can be expressed as $N = N_0\, e^{-\lambda t}$ (the variables are defined in the discussion of natural logarithms). Express this relationship in a logarithmic form using a single logarithm.
15. (8-18) If radiation output in air as a function of kVp for fixed distance, filtration, and mAs for most x-ray machines is plotted on log-log paper, the result will approximate a straight line with a slope of approximately +2. What is the relationship between the output and kVp?

Problems related to this chapter

16. What is the common logarithm of 10,000?
17. What is $\log(^4/_B)$ in terms of $\log(^B/_A)$?
18. What is ln 15?
19. Evaluate log 0.052.
20. Find x if $\log x = 1.73$.
21. Find y if $\ln y = 3.3$.
22. Use logarithms to evaluate $(2.5)^{3.2}$ as a single decimal number.
23. What is the common logarithm of the fifth root of 10?
24. Solve the equation $I = I_0 e^{-\mu x}$ for x.
25. Solve the equation $\lambda_0 e^{-\lambda_0 t} = \lambda_1 e^{-\lambda_1 t}$ for t.

Objective questions

26. The value of $\log_{10} 100$ is:
    a. -2 d. 1
    b. 0   e. 2
    c. 0.693
27. If $N = A \times B$, log N is equal to:
    a. $\log A + \log B$
    b. $\log A - \log B$
    c. $\log A \times \log B$
    d. $\log A/\log B$
    e. None of these
28. If $\log_{10} x = 0$, x is:
    a. 0   d. 10
    b. 0.1   e. ≈ 3.16
    c. 1
29. The expression $(\log A - \log B)$ is equal to:
    a. $\log(^B/_A)$ d. $\log(A + B)$
    b. $\log(^A/_B)$ e. None of these
    c. $\log(A - B)$

30. The natural logarithm of $e^{-\mu x}$ is:
    a. $-\mu x$ d. 2.30
    b. μx e. 0
    c. $^1/_\mu$
31. The formula $I = I_0 10^{-D}$ can be solved for D as:
    a. $D = I_0 10^{-I}$
    b. $D = I\,10^{-I_0}$
    c. $D = \log \dfrac{I_0}{I}$
    d. $\log D = \dfrac{I}{I_0}$
    e. $D = \log I + \log I_0$
32. The numbers 201 and 0.201 will have the same:
    a. mantissa
    b. square root
    c. characteristic
    d. logarithm
    e. absolute value
33. On semilogarithmic paper (log scale vertical) a graph appears as a straight line with a negative slope. With K and L as positive constants, the relationship is of the form:
    a. $y = {}^K/_x + L$
    b. $y = {}^K/_{x^2} + L$
    c. $y = Ke^{-L/x}$
    d. $y = Ke^{-x/L}$

CHAPTER 9

Probability and statistics

MATHEMATICAL PROBABILITY

When I come through the door dripping little puddles on the carpet and someone asks me, "Is it raining outside?" the answer is rather obvious. The situation is different if I'm asked, "Will it rain tomorrow?" or "Will a patient's pneumonia be cured by a course of penicillin?" or "Will the next patient who calls Dr. Jones be a man?" Although the answers to these questions will eventually—by tomorrow, in a week, in an hour—*have* to be either affirmative or negative, at this moment they can only be "maybe." Yet in mathematical terms all such situations, those that have at least two distinct outcomes, can be handled by the concept of *probability*.

CHANCE AND RANDOMNESS. The relative *chance* or probability of an outcome can be expressed in several ways. For example, if a blindfolded man gropes for one of ten names in a hat, the likelihood of his pulling out a certain one, say Smith, can be called $1/10$, 0.1, 10%, or "one in ten." In the language of probability the first two terms are the accepted forms; everyday speech prefers "percent" or "one in ten."

Here are some other terms used when dealing with probability: A single episode, measurement, or trial is called an *event*. Examples are the flipping of a coin, an estimate of the amount of change in my pocket or of the number of patients currently admitted to the hospital, and the "educated guess" about whether a patient has a specific disease. The result associated with a certain event, be it a yes, a no, or a specific value, is called the *outcome*. Every event *must* have an outcome; if there is no outcome, there was no event. For example, if a flipped coin drops to the floor and rolls out of sight, we do not consider the flip complete or usable. The postulate that every true event (by definition) must have an outcome leads to the conclusion that the probabilities of all possible outcomes add up to unity. For example, in the names-in-a-hat situation, each of the ten names had a probability of $1/10$ of being pulled. The ten tenths, of course, add up to one.

Rule 9-1. *The sum of the probabilities of all distinct outcomes is one.*

This rule has several useful consequences. If a particular outcome is a *certainty*, that is, only one outcome is possible, its probability is one. If all the names in that hat had been Smith, for example, the outcome would be a certainty, its probability, one.

Rule 9-2. *The probability for an outcome that is certain is one.*

Conversely, if an outcome had no chance at all, if it is *impossible,* its probability is zero.

Rule 9-3. *The probability of an impossible outcome is zero.*

Obviously, no probability analysis is needed for events whose outcomes are either certain or impossible. We will be concerned here only with events whose outcomes are possible but not certain—where, in other words, the probability will lie between zero and one.

Sources of randomness. Before delving into its mathematics, perhaps we should ask *what determines probability.* Physics tells us that all events in nature are subject to physical laws, that their outcomes are therefore dictated by these laws and that, by correct application of these laws, we should be able to determine these outcomes. If, for instance, a coin of a certain weight is flipped with a certain force, the laws of physics should tell us how many times it will turn over before it comes to rest on a certain surface and, therefore, which side will be up. Likewise, the sex of an unborn child has been determined by certain natural laws, although the parents may not yet know if it is going to be a boy or a girl. How does chance enter into these situations? One source of uncertainty is *lack of information.* Whereas the sex of Dr. Jones' next caller is probably no secret, Dr. Jones does not know this information at this moment. Part of the chance element in flipping a coin comes from this lack of information; in fact, we usually do not even observe which side of the coin is up before the flip. In these examples we lack only one element of information, but in others many such elements may be needed to specify the complete situation. For instance, a complete census of the American population would require so many details that they could not be recorded or stored even by the largest computer system. This points out a second cause of uncertainty. A situation may contain so *much information* that it is better to work with averages, typical or representative samples, or some other form of simplification. In doing this, some information may be discarded or not obtained to the extent available.

A third source of uncertainty lies in the fundamental *inability to gather information* from discrete physical systems. In physics this is called the "uncertainty principle." Its workings are most evident in systems consisting of a very small number of atoms, and occasionally in much larger entities such as a human organism or an x-ray film.

Surprisingly, problems of uncertainty arising from all three sources can be handled by the same mathematics, provided we can ensure *randomness.*

A random system is one in which the outcomes have not been *biased* in any way that is not accounted for. In games of chance involving cards, coins, roulette wheels, etc., a random event is often called an "honest" event. Non-random outcomes will result if we use a two-headed coin, weighted dice, an ace up the sleeve, or a warped roulette wheel. Many medical and biological experiments have been defective because the subjects were not randomly selected, for example, when more curable patients received the treatment that the researcher is trying to prove superior. More often than not such bias is unintentional, and sometimes it is unavoidable. The situation is not random if it is biased in any way that cannot be properly accounted for in the outcome probabilities. In the rest of this chapter it will be assumed that all the events are random.

Predictions and models. In probability, as in other applications of mathematics, extensive use is made of *models*. A model need not be a perfect fit to the real situation; often a simplification will do. For example, the sex of babies is often assumed to be equally divided when, in fact, there are several percent more male babies than female. For most purposes this approximation is adequate; a cigar manufacturer would make equal numbers of bands saying "it's a girl" and "it's a boy." On the other hand, it is important to realize that models often contain approximations that may be important. *Probability predictions* are no better than the underlying model; faulty approximations will lead to incorrect conclusions in probability as in other predictive sciences.

Law of large populations. What is the meaning of probabilities? Theoretically, a single event may produce any outcome that has a nonzero probability. This theorem has lead some people to the idea that "anything is possible." Conversely, if an outcome does not have a probability of one, it may not happen. Thus although 99% of the patients with a certain disease may be cured, there is a chance that one particular patient under treatment now will not be cured. Probability can do more for us than simply categorizing events as impossible, possible, and certain. The finer distinctions and precise probability projections become important when not one but many events are viewed. If there are enough events, all the possibility outcomes will occur, and those of higher probability will occur more often than those of lower probability. In fact, if there are n events (as long as n is large enough) and the probability of a particular outcome is p, the approximate number (N) of times this outcome will occur is pn. For example, if a coin is flipped 1,000 times, heads ($p = \frac{1}{2}$) will turn up in about 500 of these flips. Note that we say *about* 500 and not *exactly* 500. This result is due to what is often called the *law of large numbers*.

Rule 9-4. *In* n *independent repetitions of an event, an outcome of probability* p *will occur about* n × p *times.*

These repetitive events can be either sequential or coincidental in time. For example, we could toss one coin a thousand times, one thousand coins once, or ten coins one hundred times.

SINGLE EVENTS. The probability of a particular outcome is represented by the letter "p" and a subscript indicating a certain condition. For example, in a coin toss, p_h might represent the probability of a head turning up. This may also be written as $p(h)$. Capital or small letters or numerals are used to represent different outcomes. With such a notation, we can rewrite rule 9-1 for a system with n distinct outcomes.

$$p_1 + p_2 + p_3 + \ldots + p_n = 1$$

Formula 9-1

Rules 2 and 3 can be rewritten as:

$$\boxed{p \text{ (certainty)} = 1}$$ **Formula 9-2**

$$\boxed{p \text{ (impossibility)} = 0}$$ **Formula 9-3**

Formula 9-1 is useful in calculating a probability if the other probabilities are known. For example, if the probability of obtaining a head on a coin toss is $\frac{1}{2}$, the probability of obtaining a tail is $1 - \frac{1}{2}$, or $\frac{1}{2}$.

> **Example 9-1.** For a female born about 1950, the probability of eventually dying of cancer is estimated to be about 0.15. What is the probability of her dying from some other cause? Because death is a certainty, its probability is 1. Thus the probability of death from other causes is $1 - 0.15$ or 0.85.

Calculating probabilities. In many situations the probabilities are already defined. For example, a film density of 1 is defined to mean that the probability of its transmitting a visible light photon is $\frac{1}{10}$, or in general, the probability of transmission $p_t = 10^{-D}$, where D is the density.

> **Example 9-2.** Find the probability that a photon is *not* transmitted by a film of density 1. Formula 9-1 shows that the probability of transmitting p_t and the probability of not transmitting p_x must be unity; $p_t + p_x = 1$. Since $p_t = 0.1$, p_x must equal 0.9.

> **Example 9-3.** In the single-hit model of radiobiology, the probability of a cell surviving a dose (D) of radiation is $p_s = e^{-D/D_0}$. D_0 is a constant (known as D-zero, or D_{37}). What is the probability of a cell surviving a dose $D = 2D_0$? Substituting $2D_0$ for D we obtain $p_s = e^{-2} \cong 0.135$.

> **Example 9-4.** In the same model, what is the probability of a cell being killed (p_k) by a dose D of radiation? This is another application of formula 9-1. Since $p_s + p_k = 1$, $p_k = 1 - p_s$, or $p_k = 1 - e^{-D/D_0}$.

The law of large numbers (rule 9-4) mentioned earlier can be written as a formula:

$$\boxed{N \cong p \cdot n}$$ **Formula 9-4**

This formula can be solved for p as:

$$p \cong {}^N\!/_n$$ **Formula 9-5**

In many practical cases N and n can be determined, and from this an approximate p can be found.

Example 9-5. In one month, 6,352 persons were treated in a certain hospital's emergency room. Of these, 27 died before they were discharged. What is the probability that a person treated in that emergency room will die before discharge? The probability of $p_d \cong \dfrac{27}{6,352} = 0.0043$.

Note that in the preceding example the probability for the next month will not be exactly the same.

Example 9-6. In a study, 216 patients with symptoms suggesting embolism were given lung scans. Lung embolisms were positively confirmed in 82 of these cases. What is the probability of a confirmation of embolisms in this situation? It is $p_e = \dfrac{82}{216} = 0.4$.

The probabilities found by using the law of large numbers are determined by measurement or experiment and are often known as *empirical probabilities*.

In certain simple situations, probabilities can be determined by elementary considerations. For example, a normal coin has two sides, and on a flip either side is equally likely to turn up. Since there are two outcomes of equal probability, each outcome must have a probability of $\frac{1}{2}$.

Example 9-7. A common die (singular of dice) has six sides. Each side has an equal chance of appearing on top. What probability is there for the side showing three dots being on top? Since $p_1 = p_2 = p_3 = p_4 = p_5 = p_6$, and since $p_1 + p_2 + p_3 + p_4 + p_5 + p_6 = 1$, $p_3 = \frac{1}{6}$.

Example 9-8. A group of 15 black and 10 white mice is placed in a cage with a maze exit. Assuming that neither the black or the white mice have been trained in the maze, what is the probability that the first mouse to reach the exit is white? The probability for each mouse being first is equal, or $\frac{1}{25}$ each. Since there are 10 white mice, the probability for a white mouse is $p_w = \frac{10}{25}$, or 0.4.

These examples represent particularly simple cases where probabilities can be calculated. If an event has n outcomes and *each is equally likely*, the probability of each outcome is $\frac{1}{n}$ or

$$\boxed{p = \frac{1}{n}}$$

Formula 9-6

The simple models considered so far consist of individual items of equal probability. The key to determining the probabilities has been this equality.

The situation is more difficult if it involves probabilities that are in known proportions or are proportional to some known quantity. Common quantities for this proportionality are length, area, volume, time, and energy.

Example 9-9. Assume that the 15 black mice in the last example have been trained and are now each twice as likely to be first through the maze as any of the 10 white mice. What is the probability now that a white mouse is first through the maze? Call the probability for an individual white mouse p_w and for an individual black mouse $p_b = 2p_w$. Adding all the probabilities, $15p_b + 10p_w = 1$, or $30p_w + 10p_w = 1$. Solving this latter equation for p_w gives $p_w = \frac{1}{40}$. Since there are 10 white mice, the probability for the first mouse being white is $\frac{10}{40} = 0.25$.

Example 9-10. A nearsighted person tries to hit a wall with a rock from a great distance. On the wall are a number of windows 1 m high and $\frac{1}{2}$ m wide. Their centers are placed every 2 m horizontally and every 3 m vertically (Fig. 9-1). What is the chance that the rock will hit a window? Each window can be considered to sit in an area of the wall measuring 2×3 m, or 6 m². The window itself is 0.5×1 m, or 0.5 m². The rock is equally likely to fall on any portion of the wall. Of its total

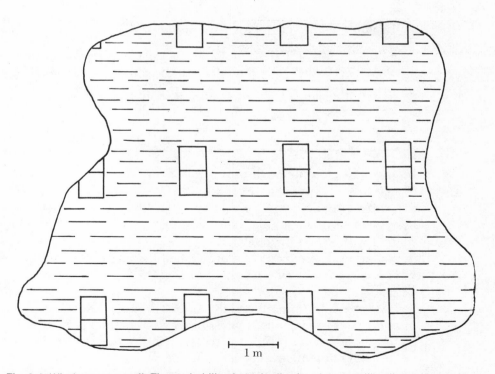

1 m

Fig. 9-1. Windows on a wall. The probability that a badly aimed stone will strike a window is the ratio of the area of the windows to the total wall area.

area, $^{0.5}/_6$, or $^1/_{12}$, of the wall is window; hence the probability of the rock hitting a window is $^1/_{12}$.

As an experiment you can take a pencil, close your eyes, and stab at Fig. 9-1. Record the stab as a hit or a miss on the window. Repeat this at least fifty times. What empirical probability do you find for striking a window?

For the problem of a point projectile striking a target of a certain area (A_t) embedded in a larger region of area (A_T) the probability can be written as follows:

$$p = A_t/A_T \qquad \qquad \textbf{Formula 9-7}$$

As in the preceding example the target area can be distributed over several targets.

> **Example 9-11.** A square centimeter of a certain metal foil contains 3×10^{18} atoms. The cross section of each atomic nucleus is 2×10^{-24} cm². What is the probability that an incident particle will strike a nucleus? The probability is the ratio of the total cross-sectional area of the nuclei to the area of the foil. This is $3 \times 10^{18} \times \dfrac{2 \times 10^{-24}}{1.0}$, or $p = 6 \times 10^{-6}$.

> **Example 9-12.** A metal foil containing $\dfrac{5 \times 10^{19} \text{ atoms}}{\text{cm}^2}$ is placed in a neutron beam. Experimental measurement shows that 1 neutron in 100,000 interacts with a nucleus in the foil. What is the cross section (σ) of the nuclei in the foil? $5 \times 10^{19} \times \sigma/1 = \dfrac{1}{100,000}$, or $\sigma = 2 \times 10^{-25}$ cm².

The preceding examples of probability associated with area assume that the projectile is a point. Sometimes a finite area projectile is used. For example, if a coin is dropped onto a checker board, it may lie completely within a square or on one or more of the lines dividing the squares. The effective area of the target will be less than the actual target area if the coin is to lie entirely within the target. If the coin need only touch the target, the effective area is larger. These two cases are illustrated in Fig. 9-2.

> **Example 9-13.** A marble of diameter 1.4 cm is thrown against a fence composed of wire mesh made of wires 0.2 cm thick placed every 10 cm in a square pattern. What is the probability that the marble will pass through without striking a wire? The area of each square is 100 cm². The area that the center of the marble can pass through so that the periphery will not touch a wire is $= 10 - 1.4 - 0.2 = 8.4$ cm on a

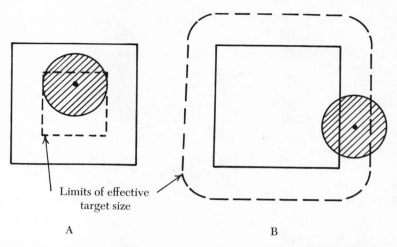

Fig. 9-2. Effective target areas for finite projectiles. In this case the target is represented by the square shown with the solid line; the projectile is indicated by the crosshatched circle. In case A a hit is scored only if the projectile lands entirely within the target; this restricts the center of the projectile to the small square outlined with the dashed line. In case B the projectile need only touch the target; in this case the effective area is much larger than the area of the target alone.

side, or 71 cm². Thus the probability of the marble passing through the fence without hitting a wire is $^{71}/_{100} = 0.71$.

MULTIPLE EVENTS. The outcome of a single event can be expressed by a single parameter. If more than one parameter is required to specify the results, this is a *multiple event*. For example, the determination of a patient's age and sex is a multiple event.

For conceptual purposes it is convenient to consider these constituent events as occurring in some sort of sequence. In multiple events we are usually interested in the probability (*P*) of the overall outcome. Thus a model for production of a bad film might consider the probability of each of the events of manufacture, storage, placement in cassette, exposure techniques, and processing. From an analysis of the probability of the single events the overall probability of a bad film could be calculated.

Discrete outcomes. First, consider a situation consisting of two single events. The overall outcome consists of two single outcomes. For convenience we will restrict ourselves to those cases where there is no ambiguity in the overall outcome and the outcome of the single event. That is, from the overall outcome, the separate outcomes can be found and vice versa. For example, if patients are distinguished by age (say less than 16 years is pediatric) and by disease (infectious or not), specifying the overall distinction specifies the individual distinctions.

For the time let us further restrict our case to situations where the two single events have two outcomes each, say A and $\overline{A}$ (the bar in this case of discrete outcomes is read as "not") for the first event, and B and $\overline{B}$ for the second. Thus there are four overall outcomes: (1) A and B, (2) A and $\bar{B}$, (3) $\bar{A}$ and B, (4) $\bar{A}$ and $\bar{B}$.

The several probabilities that may concern us here are the single event probabilities p_A, $p_{\bar{A}}$, p_B, and $p_{\bar{B}}$ and the multiple event probabilities $p(A$ and $B)$, $p(\bar{A}$ and $B)$, etc. In addition, there are the conditional probabilities, such as $p(A|\bar{B})$, which is read "the probability of A assuming not B"; this is the probability that A occurs once we know that B has not occurred. As an example, consider the probabilities of a child having brown eyes or being a boy. Use A to represent brown eyes, $\bar{A}$ for eyes not brown, B for a boy, and $\bar{B}$ for a girl (= not boy). The symbol $p(A$ and $\bar{B})$ is the probability of having a girl with brown eyes, whereas $p(A|\bar{B})$ is the probability of having brown eyes *if* the child is a girl.

For our set of events, formula 9-1 must apply in several ways. For example, all outcomes must have either A or $\bar{A}$. Thus:

$$p(A) + p(\bar{A}) = 1$$

The probabilities of all outcomes must total 1:

$$p(A \text{ and } B) + p(\bar{A} \text{ and } B) + p(A \text{ and } \bar{B}) + p(\bar{A} \text{ and } \bar{B}) = 1$$

And if we assume one of the single outcomes, say B, then:

$$p(A|B) + p(\bar{A}|B) = 1$$

The outcome $(A$ and $B)$ assumes both the outcome A and the outcome B. The probability of this $p(A$ and $B)$ can be broken into two pieces—the probability of B, or $p(B)$, and the probability of A assuming B, or $p(A|B)$. These are combined by multiplication as usual for combining probabilities of different events:

$$p(A \text{ and } \bar{B}) = p(A|B) \times p(\bar{B})$$

$$p(A) = p(A \text{ and } B) + p(A \text{ and } \bar{B})$$

Example 9-14. In a certain class of 20 technology students, 7 males and 7 females expect to become radiographers, the 4 other males and 2 females expect to work in therapy. Use F and M for sex differentiation and R and T for professional intent. Find $p(F)$ directly and also by using $p(F) = p(F$ and $R)$ and $p(F$ and $T)$. Since there are 9 females out of 20 students, $p(F) = 9/20 = 0.45$. Also, $p(F$ and $R) = 7/20 = 0.35$ and $p(F$ and $T) = 2/20 = 0.1$. Thus $p(F) = 0.35 + 0.1 = 0.45$ again.

Independence and causality. Single events are *independent* if the outcome of one event has no influence on the outcome of the other. For example, experiments could utilize guinea pigs that have either black or brown and either curly or straight coats; if hair color and hair texture are independent, the probability of curly hair is the same for black and for brown guinea pigs. Or, in general, if the two single events are independent:

$$\boxed{p(A) \ = \ p(A|B) \ = \ p(A|\bar{B})}$$ **Formula 9-8**

Example 9-15. Are the events (sex and professional intent) listed in example 9-14 independent? For this to be true, $p(F) = p(F|T) = p(F|R)$ and $p(M) = p(M|R) = p(M|T)$, but $p(F) = 0.45$, $p(F|R) = 0.50$, and $p(F|T) = 0.33$, while $p(M) = 0.55$, $p(M|R) = 0.50$, and $p(M|T) = 0.67$. Thus the two events are not independent.

If events are not independent, they *correlate*. In examples 9-14 and 9-15 there is a correlation between sex and professional preference. In the sample class males show a greater preference for therapy than is shown by females. If events correlate, there are two possible reasons. One is a simple fluctuation, which is often found in a small sample. The other is some built-in difference, or *causal* relationship. Statistics is primarily useful in determining whether fluctuations can be ruled out as a cause of a given correlation. Put another way, statistics is used to demonstrate the existence of a causal relationship.

If events are independent, the outcomes are readily predicted. In general:

$$p(A \text{ and } B) \ = \ p(A|B) \ \times \ p(B)$$

If A and B are outcomes of independent events:

$$p(A|B) \ = \ p(A)$$

or

$$p(A \text{ and } B) \ = \ p(A) \ \times \ p(B)$$ **Formula 9-9**

Example 9-16. Assume that the sex of each child in a family is independent and $p(F) = p(M) = \frac{1}{2}$. What is the probability of a two-child family having two children of the same sex? This probability, labeled as $p(\text{same}) = p(F \text{ and } F) + p(M \text{ and } M)$; $p(F \text{ and } F) = p(F)p(F) = (\frac{1}{2}) \times (\frac{1}{2}) = \frac{1}{4}$, and similarly $p(M \text{ and } M) = \frac{1}{4}$. Thus the probability of having two children of the same sex is $\frac{1}{2}$.

Probability trees. For multiple events that are not independent a representation that is often convenient is a *probability tree*. A typical example is shown in Fig. 9-3. The tree begins at the left and branches out to the right. The branches from a particular apex represent the conditional probabilities at that point. The probability for any particular end point is found from the product of all the branches from the start to the end point. For example, the chance that a patient will be assigned to room 2 and technician B and that a good film will result is $p(2,B,\text{good}) = 0.3 \times 0.3 \times 0.9 = 0.081$.

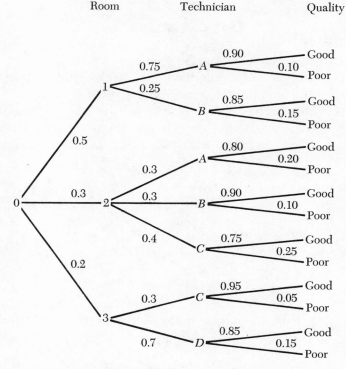

Fig. 9-3. A probability tree representing the assignment of a patient for a radiograph in a department with 3 rooms and 4 technicians.

Example 9-17. What is the chance of a patient being assigned to room 1 with technician *A* and also having a good film? This is 0.5 × 0.75 × 0.9 = 0.34.

Not only can the probabilities of single final outcomes be calculated in this manner and the explicit conditional probabilities read off, but also, by grouping outcomes, various other probabilities can be found. For example, in the tree of Fig. 9-3 we can figure the probability of a good picture for any given patient by adding all the good outcomes.

Example 9-18. What is the chance that a patient will be assigned to technician *A*? $p(1,A) = 0.5 \times 0.75 = 0.375$, $p(2,A) = 0.3 \times 0.3 = 0.090$, and $p(3,A) = 0$; also $p(A) = p(1,A) + p(2,A) + p(3, A) = 0.375 + 0.090 + 0 = 0.465$.

Permutations and combinations. A common situation in probability is the distribution of a certain number of items at a number of specified sites. For example, a class of six students enters a room with eight chairs; how many different ways can these students sit? From such considerations we can use formula 9-6 to calculate the probability of a given arrangement assuming that the seating is random.

The simplest case is for a number of items situated in the same number of sites. Any possible configuration can be made from any other by selective interchange, or *permutation*. The number of different configurations is known as the *number of permutations*.

The number of permutations for a given number is readily calculated by a simple thought process. Consider as an example four sites for four items. The items will be placed at the sites one at a time for convenience. The first item can be placed at any of the four different sites. There are only three sites at which to place the second item, since the first item already occupies one site; thus there are 4×3 or 12 ways to place the first two items. Only 2 sites remain available for the third item; once this is placed there is only one site, or no choice, for the last item. Overall, the number of permutations of four items, sometimes known as $P(r)$ is:

$$P(4) = 4 \times 3 \times 2 \times 1 = 24$$

For a general number of items and sites (k) the number of permutations is:

$$P(k) = k(k - 1)\,(k - 2) \ldots (3)\,(2)\,1$$

Because this special product appears frequently, it is given a special notation and name:

$$\boxed{P(k) = k!}$$

Formula 9-10

where $k!$ is called k *factorial* and is defined as follows:

$$\boxed{k! = k(k - 1)\,(k - 2) \ldots (3)\,(2)\,1}$$

Formula 9-11

Example 9-19. What is 5!? It is $5 \times 4 \times 3 \times 2 \times 1 = 120$.

Example 9-20. What is the probability that a group of five items will be arranged in five positions in a certain way by random chance? There are 5!, or 120, possible arrangements. Each arrangement is equally likely; the probability of any one arrangement is $1/120$.

Frequently there are more items than places. If the number of items is n and the number of places is k, then, in a manner analogous to the one used to find the number of permutations, it can be shown that there are $(n)\,(n - 1) \ldots (n - k + 2)\,(n - k + 1) = \dfrac{n!}{(n - k)!}$ different arrangements possible. Note that this relationship is consistent with formula 9-10 for $n = k$ provided 0! is defined as being equal to 1.

If we are concerned only with which of the n items appear in the k sites but not the arrangements in the sites, we have what is called the number of *combinations*. Since the items in the k sites can be permuted $k!$ ways, the number of combinations of n items in k sites is:

$$C^n_k = \frac{n!}{(n-k)!\,(k)!}$$
Formula 9-12

> **Example 9-21.** A certain radiology department has 15 rooms. If three rooms are kept running every evening, how many different combinations of three are possible? This is a direct application of formula 9-16 for C^{15}_{13}; this is $\dfrac{15!}{12! \times 3!} = \dfrac{15 \times 14 \times 13}{3 \times 2 \times 1} = 455$.

PROBABILITY DISTRIBUTIONS

When there are a great many possible outcomes or when the outcomes are on a continuous or nearly continuous scale it is frequently convenient to use a probability *distribution*. The best-known distribution is the *normal* or bell-shaped distribution widely used in handling test scores. We can use the distribution to ascertain the probability of a particular outcome.

THEORETICAL DISTRIBUTIONS. If a theoretical model of a random system exists, the probability theory developed earlier in this chapter, or an extension of it, can be used to derive a theoretical distribution. For example, if the model of equal probability of the sex of children is used, a family of seven children has probabilities of $1/128$, $7/128$, $21/128$, $35/128$, $35/128$, $21/128$, $7/128$, and $1/128$ for 0,1,2,3,4,5,6, and 7 children of one sex, respectively. This distribution is plotted in Fig. 9-4.

When the possibility of a large number of outcomes exists, the detailed probability of a given outcome is often not desired. Rather, a few statistical parameters are often more useful descriptors of the situation. The parameters that will be most useful will represent the average magnitude and the spread of the distribution. The *average magnitude* is usually given in terms of the *algebraic mean*, frequently called the *average* or *mean*; occasionally the geometric mean is useful. For the example in Fig. 9-4 the mean, 3.5, is readily seen from the symmetry. Two other measures of the quantity are the median and the mode; the *median* is the quantity so situated that the probability of being above it is $1/2$.

> **Example 9-22.** What is the probability of an outcome being below the median? This is one minus the probability of being above, or $1 - 1/2 = 1/2$.

The most likely outcome is called the *mode*. For a symmetrical distribution such as in Fig. 9-4 the mean, mode, and median are all equal.

Another parameter of great importance is the *spread of the distribution*.

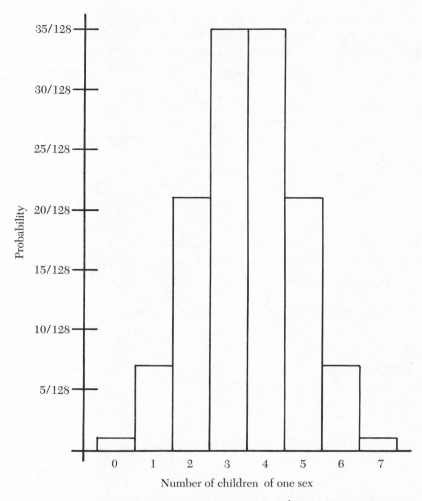

Fig. 9-4. The probability distribution of sexes in a family with 7 children.

This is useful in predicting whether outcomes differing from the average are reasonably likely or not.

EXPERIMENTAL DISTRIBUTIONS. The result of an experiment (event) repeated a number of times will be a distribution of results (outcomes). If the experiment were exactly repeated, the result in most cases would differ from the initial result. However, if the number of trials is large, we would expect the average result to be very close to the average result of another large number of trials.

Unlike the theoretical model, which will produce an exact probability for a specific outcome, the *experimental distribution* is not constant. The average value and the spread are likely to be similar from one experiment to the next.

Mean and standard deviation. The mean of several quantities is found by summing the quantities and dividing by the number of quantities. For example, the mean of 3, 5, and 10 is $\dfrac{(3 + 5 + 10)}{3} = 6$.

Example 9-23. The five technicians in a certain nuclear medicine facility performed 8, 12, 9, 13, and 6 scans, respectively, on a certain day. What was the average (mean) number of scans produced? This is $\frac{(8 + 12 + 9 + 13 + 6)}{5} = \frac{48}{5} = 9.6$.

Formally, we can call the quantities $x_1, x_2, \ldots x_i$ in general. For n quantities the mean is:

$$\bar{x} = \frac{(x_1 + x_2 \ldots \ldots x_n)}{n} = \frac{1}{n} \sum_{i=1}^{n} x_i$$

Formula 9-13

The bar over numerical quantities means average. The sigma indicates that the sum is to be taken; the $i = 1$ shows that i has the value 1 for the first term, whereas the n at the top indicates that n is the subscript of the last term. The entire symbol $\sum_{i=1}^{n}$ is read "the sum from $i = 1$ to $i = n$." This is a common notation.

The preceding definition of the mean assumes that each quantity is equally likely. If, however, some quantities are more likely than others—an example is the distribution of Fig. 9-4—a *weight* (f_i) is assigned to each x_i and the formula for the mean becomes:

$$\bar{x} = \frac{(f_1 x_1 + f_2 x_2 + \ldots \ldots + f_n x_n)}{(f_1 + f_2 + \ldots \ldots + f_n)} = \frac{\left(\sum_{i=1}^{n} f_i x_i\right)}{\left(\sum_{i=1}^{n} f_i\right)}$$

Formula 9-14

If the weights are probabilities, the mean may be called the *expectation value*.

Example 9-24. Use formula 9-10 to verify the previous statement concerning the average of the distribution of Fig. 9-4. The sum $\sum_{i=1}^{n} f_i x_i =$

$(\frac{1}{128})0 + (\frac{7}{128})1 + (\frac{21}{128})2 + (\frac{35}{128})3 + (\frac{35}{128})4 + (\frac{21}{128})5 + (\frac{7}{128})6$

$+ (\frac{1}{128})7 = \frac{(7 + 42 + 105 + 140 + 105 + 42 + 7)}{128} = \frac{448}{128} =$

3.5; the sum $\sum_{i=1}^{n} f_i = \frac{1}{128} + \frac{7}{128} + \frac{21}{128} + \frac{35}{128} + \frac{35}{128} + \frac{21}{128} + \frac{7}{128} + \frac{1}{128}$

$= \frac{128}{128} = 1$ as we expect for a proper probability distribution. Thus $\bar{x} = 3.5$.

In an experimental situation, measurements are made to ascertain approximate values for the underlying hypothesis. As the experiment is repeated more and more times, the experimental statistical parameters will get closer and closer to the theoretical values.

The *standard deviation* is a measure of the spread of a distribution above and below the theoretical average. For a theoretical distribution calculated from a model, the standard deviation is defined as the square root of the average square deviation from the theoretical mean. We will use the notation $\langle \mu \rangle$ to represent the theoretical mean. Then the standard deviation for equally likely outcomes, represented by the small Greek letter sigma, is:

Formula 9-15

$$\sigma = \sqrt{\frac{[(\langle \mu \rangle - x_1)^2 + (\langle \mu \rangle - x_2)^2 + \ldots + (\langle \mu \rangle - x_n)^2]}{n}} = \sqrt{\frac{1}{n} \sum_{i=1}^{n} (\langle \mu \rangle - x_i)^2}$$

If the experimental mean $\bar{x}$ is known but the theoretical mean $\langle \mu \rangle$ is not, the experimental standard deviation can still be estimated by replacing the n in the denominator with $n - 1$:

$$\sigma \cong \sqrt{\frac{[(\bar{x} - x_1)^2 + (\bar{x} - x_2)^2 + \ldots + (\bar{x} - x_n)^2]}{(n - 1)}}$$

or

$$\sigma \cong \sqrt{\frac{1}{n - 1} \sum_{i=1}^{n} (\bar{x} - x_i)^2}$$

Formula 9-16

Example 9-25. In example 9-23 five technicians performed 8, 12, 9, 13, and 6 scans apiece. The average number of scans ($\bar{x}$) is 9.6. Find the standard deviation. The deviations are 1.6, -2.4, 0.6, -3.4, and 3.6, respectively; their squares add to 33.20. Then

$$\sigma = \sqrt{\frac{33.20}{(5-1)}} = \sqrt{8.30} \cong 2.88.$$

In simple words, the standard deviation is roughly the average deviation from the mean encountered in most measurements.

COMMON DISTRIBUTIONS. Most simple models lead to a probability distribution whose terms are the result of expanding a binomial taken to an appropriate power. This distribution is known as the *binomial* distribution. There are two specialized modifications of the binomial distribution used for a very large number of events: the normal and the Poisson distributions.

Binomial distribution. Consider the case of a radiation dose that will kill 20% of a large population of mice. That is, the probability (p) of a mouse being killed by this dose is $1/5$. The probability of it not being killed is $4/5$; call this $\bar{p}$. If we expose one mouse, its probabilities are $p + \bar{p} = 1$, which indicates that the mouse has an either/or prognosis. If two mice are exposed, each has the same p and $\bar{p}$. The combined probability of all outcomes could be written as

$(p_1 + \overline{p}_1) (p_2 + \overline{p}_2)$, since independent probabilities are multiplicative. This can be expanded to $p_1 p_2$ (both survive) $+ \overline{p}_1 p_2$ (no. 1 dies, no. 2 survives) $+ p_1 \overline{p}_2$ (no. 1 survives, no. 2 dies) $+ \overline{p}_1 \overline{p}_2$ (both die). If we are not interested in the individual mice, then the subscripts can be dropped, yielding $(p + \overline{p}) \times (p + \overline{p})$ $= p^2 + p\overline{p} + \overline{p}p + \overline{p}^2 = p^2 + 2p\overline{p} + \overline{p}^2 = (p + \overline{p})^2$. The power 2 appears because there are two individuals.

> **Example 9-26.** In this case what is the probability that one mouse is killed and one survives? This is the term containing $p\overline{p}$, which is $2p\overline{p}$, or $2(\frac{1}{5})(\frac{4}{5}) = \frac{8}{25}$, or 0.32.

Suppose four mice were irradiated under these conditions. Then the probabilities are represented as follows:

$$(p + \overline{p})^4 = p^4 + 4p^3\overline{p} + 6p^2\overline{p}^2 + 4p\overline{p}^3 + \overline{p}^4$$

For a particular outcome—say 2 killed and 2 survive—the probability is the *binomial coefficient*, 6 in this case, multiplied by the individual probabilities to the appropriate power, or, P (2 killed, 2 survive) $= 6p^2\overline{p}^2$.

The binomial coefficients are equal to the number of combinations in that situation. That is, if there are n single events with k positive outcomes, the binomial coefficient is just $C_k^n = \dfrac{n!}{k! \, (n - k)!}$. Thus the probability of k positive outcomes in n single events is:

$$P_k^n = C_k^n \, p^k \overline{p}^{n-k} \qquad \text{Formula 9-17}$$

> **Example 9-27.** If 1,000 cells are exposed to a photon beam that has a probability of killing each cell $p = 0.999$, what is the chance that all cells are killed? (NOTE: $n = 1,000$, $k = 1,000$, and $n - k = 0$.)
>
> $$P = C\binom{1,000}{1,000} \times (0.999)^{1,000} = 1 \times 0.37 = 0.37$$
>
> Note that this means there is a probability of 0.63 for one or more cells surviving.

Properties of the binomial distribution can be derived from formula 9-17. For convenience, the results are given without derivation. The average number of positive outcomes in n events if p is the probability of a positive outcome in a single event (and $\overline{p} = 1 - p$) is given by formula 9-4 as:

$$\langle \mu \rangle = np$$

and the standard deviation is

$$\sigma = \sqrt{np\overline{p}} \qquad \text{Formula 9-18}$$

The example shown in Fig. 9-4 is a binomial distribution with $n = 7$ and $p = \bar{p} = \frac{1}{2}$. Thus $\langle \mu \rangle = 7(\frac{1}{2}) = 3.5$ as found before and

$$\sigma = \sqrt{7(\frac{1}{2})\,\frac{1}{2}} = \sqrt{\frac{7}{4}} \cong 1.32$$

Poisson distribution. If the number of single events in a multiple event becomes very large, the binomial probabilities become difficult to calculate because of the large factorials and high powers. For this reason it is frequently convenient to utilize approximate distributions where the approximations are valid.

If the number of events (n) becomes *very large*, but the probability of a positive outcome (p) is *extremely small*, so that the number of likely outcomes, $N = pn$ by formula 9-4, is *not large*, the *Poisson distribution* or "Poisson statistics" applies. These conditions are met for most practical ionizing radiation–counting situations in radiology; for example, in determining the activity of a sample there is a very large number of potential decays that could lead to counts, whereas in an actual situation only a small fraction of the nuclei actually decay during counting, and of these decays usually only a few percent actually yield counts. Also, there are many other problems of interest that will utilize Poisson statistics. These include accident and mortality statistics, mechanical breakdowns, and the incidence of certain diseases such as cancer.

In the Poisson approximation the probability of k positive outcomes in n events is:

$$P\binom{n}{k} = \frac{(np)^k\, e^{-np}}{k!} \qquad\qquad \text{Formula 9-19}$$

Example 9-28. A tumor containing 10^9 cells is irradiated so that the probability of any single cell surviving is 10^{-10}. What are the probabilities $p(0)$, of 0 cells surviving, $p(1)$, of 1 cell surviving, and $p(2)$, of 2 cells surviving? These are $p\binom{10^9}{0}$, $p\binom{10^9}{1}$ and $p\binom{10^9}{2}$ respectively.

$$p(0) = \frac{(0.1)^0\, e^{-0.1}}{0!} \cong 0.905$$

$$p(1) = \frac{(0.1)^1\, e^{-0.1}}{1!} \cong 0.090$$

$$p(2) = \frac{(0.1)^2\, e^{-0.1}}{2!} \cong 0.005$$

Of greater importance than the individual probabilities of formula 9-19 is the standard deviation of this distribution, which is:

$$\boxed{\sigma = \sqrt{np} = \sqrt{N}} \qquad\qquad \text{Formula 9-20}$$

We emphasize here that N is the average number of positive outcomes—the same as $\langle x \rangle$ or $\overline{x}$.

> **Example 9-29.** A certain large hospital normally has about 25 employees on sick leave at any one time. What is the standard deviation of this number? The standard deviation, $\sigma = \sqrt{25} = 5$.

> **Example 9-30.** The information density in a 1 cm square of a certain scan is 800 counts/cm². What is the standard deviation in counts for this square? It is $\sqrt{800} \cong 28$ counts.

The detailed application of Poisson statistics to "counting" will be considered later in this chapter.

Normal distribution. When the number of single events (n) composing a multiple event becomes *very large* and the probability of a single event (p) is *large* enough that $N = np$ is *not a small* value, the binomial distribution becomes a symmetrical humped distribution centered around N. In this case the convenient approximate distribution is the *normal distribution*. This distribution is also known by the names Gaussian, error function, or bell-shaped distribution.

It is common practice to "renormalize" the normal curve, usually by placing the average at zero. Thus the only consideration is the spread of the function as represented by the standard deviation. A Gaussian function plotted on the scale of the standard deviation is shown in Fig. 9-5. The distribution is represented by a smooth curve because many contiguous values are included. When used in the manner shown in Fig. 9-5 the curve obeys the following form:

$$y = \frac{1}{\sqrt{2\pi}} e^{-x^2/2}$$

Formula 9-21

Here y is the relative probability and x is the deviation from the average divided by the standard deviation. The normal distribution is rarely used in this way. The customary use is for a range of values; for example, we might want to know the probability of being *within* one standard deviation, that is, between -1σ and $+1\sigma$ in the example in Fig. 9-5, of the average (0).

In this case we are interested in the *area* under the curve for the range in question. For this distribution these areas cannot be expressed as a simple function. Values can be found in any standard set of mathematics tables. For many purposes three values are commonly used and should be remembered:

Area $(-\sigma$ to $+\sigma) = 0.68$

Area $(-2\sigma$ to $+2\sigma) = 0.95$

Area $(-3\sigma$ to $+3\sigma) = 0.997$

This means that the probability of being within 1 standard deviation of the

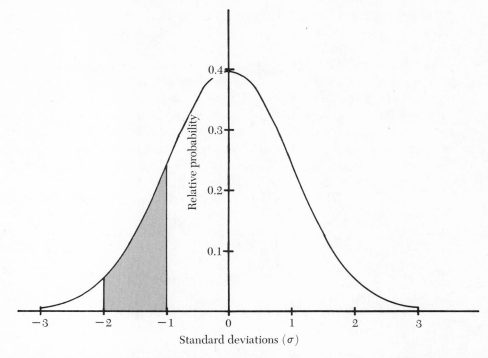

Fig. 9-5. The normal distribution. The area under the entire curve is equal to 1. For any range of the standard deviation, the probability that the outcome of an event lies between two limits (e.g., −2, −1) corresponds to the area under the curve bounded by the two limits.

mean in a normal distribution is 0.68 (roughly $\frac{2}{3}$), the probability of being within 2 standard deviations is 0.95, and the probability of being within 3 standard deviations is 0.997.

> **Example 9-31.** What is the probability of a result being beyond 1 standard deviation in a normal distribution? Since the probability of being within 1 standard deviation is 0.68, the probability of being beyond is $1 - 0.68 = 0.32$.

> **Example 9-32.** What is the probability of obtaining a result between the mean μ and the value $\mu + 2\sigma$? Since the normal distribution is symmetrical, the area under the curve from $\mu - 2\sigma$ to μ is equal to the area under the curve from μ to $\mu + 2\sigma$. Thus the area (probability) from μ to $\mu + 2\sigma = (\frac{1}{2})0.95 = 0.48$.

APPLICATIONS OF STATISTICS

There are two main *applications of statistics* to practical problems. The first is predicting the outcome of experiments such as measurements, trials, and polls in systems assumed to have random fluctuations in which some of the statistical parameters (for example, μ and σ) are known from theory or experiment. The second is estimating the chance that two results of matched experiments differ in a significant way.

COUNTING STATISTICS. A series of problems in radiology deal with statistics of a type commonly called *counting statistics*. These are generally of two types. One is the pulse counting associated with detectors such as Geiger-Mueller (GM) and scintillation detectors; in these systems a certain number of "counts" is scored by the detector. The other system is the two-dimensional counting system of which x-ray films and scintillation scans or camera images are examples; in this case we can speak of the number of counts in a small area, or "picture element," sometimes known as a *pixel*. In the simplest counting schemes the fluctuations are determined almost exclusively by the number of quanta detected; this is the count in pulse counting systems. In a system in which the number of quanta increases at some stage of image manipulation—in an intensifying screen or a fluoroscopic image intensifier for example —the statistics are determined by that level of image containing the fewest quanta; in the case of intensifying screens this level is the level of photons absorbed in the screens.

All but a very few of the counting situations match the approximations for both the Poisson and the normal distributions. As a result we can use the Poisson standard deviation formula (9-20) $\sigma = \sqrt{N}$ and the probabilities of the normal distribution.

> **Example 9-33.** A certain long-lived radioactive source is counted for 1 min. This results in 2,500 counts. If the count is repeated, what is the chance that the result will *not* be between 2,400 and 2,600? For this case $\sigma = \sqrt{2,500} = 50$; 2,400 is 100, or 2σ less than 2,500, and 2,600 is 2σ more. Thus if the second count is outside the 2,400 to 2,600 range, it is beyond 2σ; the probability of this is about $1 - 0.95 = 0.05$, or $\frac{1}{20}$.

Several common variants on the simple application of the standard deviation are used. First, the standard deviation (σ) is often expressed as a fraction of the counts; this is σ/N. Since $\sigma = \sqrt{N}$, the *fractional deviation* is expressed in the following formula:

$$\frac{\sigma}{N} = \frac{\sqrt{N}}{N} = \frac{1}{\sqrt{N}}$$

Formula 9-22

In some cases this ratio is expressed as a percent and is known as "percent statistics"; for 1% statistics $\sigma/N = 1/\sqrt{N} = 0.01$, then $N = \dfrac{1}{(0.01)^2} = 10,000$.

Example 9-34. How many counts are needed for 5% statistics? Here $0.05 = \dfrac{1}{\sqrt{N}}$, or $N = \dfrac{1}{(0.05)^2} = 400$.

If counts are recorded in rate units such as counts per minute (cpm), then the counting rate will have the same fractional deviation as the entire count. It is necessary to find the standard deviation for the total counts (the product of the count rate and time).

Example 9-35. A certain sample is counted for 10 min. The result is a count rate of 165 cpm. Express this count rate with an uncertainty equal to 1 standard deviation. Note we cannot simply take the square root of 165. The total number of counts is 1,650; the standard deviation of this is $\sqrt{1,650} \cong 40.6$, or, as a fractional deviation, 0.0246. The fractional deviation of the count rate will be the same—0.0246. Thus the standard deviation will be the product of the fractional deviation and 165; it is 4.1. The count rate is correctly expressed as 165 ± 4.1 cpm.

With a rate meter of the type often found on a GM counter, the total of counts used for calculating the standard deviation is the product of the count rate and "response time." The needle of such a meter can be expected to fluctuate by roughly 2σ on either side of the true rate.

Example 9-36. A Geiger survey meter with a 4 sec response time is averaging 400 cpm in a constant radiation field. What is the range of oscillations of the needle on the meter? In 4 sec, $400 \times \frac{4}{60} = 26.7$ counts are anticipated; the fractional deviation will be $\dfrac{1}{\sqrt{26.7}} \cong \dfrac{1}{5.16}$ $\cong 0.194$. One standard deviation around 400 cpm would be $400 \times 0.194 = 77.5$ cpm; 2 standard deviations will be 155 cpm. The range of the meter needle will be from about 245 to 555 cpm.

Example 9-37. A flood field view on a scanner is recorded to an information density of 800 counts/cm². What is the information density uncertainty (1 standard deviation) for pixels of 1 cm², 0.25cm², and 0.04 cm²? These pixels will average 800, 200, and 32 counts respectively; the fractional deviations for these three cases are 0.035, 0.071, and 0.18. Thus the information densities are 800 ± 28 cm^{-2}, 800 ± 57 cm^{-2}, and 800 ± 141 cm^{-2}.

Statistical tests. It can be seen from some of the examples in the preceding sections that two seemingly identical measurements will not necessarily yield exactly the same results. What can be said of two measurements of situations that might be different? For example, suppose a radioactive sample is counted as yielding 675 counts in 1 min. Ten minutes later this same sample, when counted again for 1 min, yields 647 counts. Are we seeing decay of a relatively short half-life sample? Because these numbers represent a change of about 1 standard deviation between the two counts, we can expect deviations this large to occur by chance alone about one third of the time. On the other hand, the results are consistent with a decay of 4% between the two measurements. Thus we are left with a dilemma that cannot be resolved without more data.

An important question in many measurements is whether the results in two cases are different enough to indicate a difference in the basic situations. We call such a difference a *significant difference*. Differences that are small enough that they could easily be a statistical fluctuation are called *nonsignificant*. The usual or *null hypothesis* is one that assumes there is no difference. A change is probably just a fluctuation if it is nonsignificant; however, a nonsignificant difference is not proof that the difference is only a fluctuation.

How significant is significant? In a system with fluctuations, large, unlikely variations will occur from time to time. What fraction of the time are we willing to accept these fluctuations as a significant difference? As a practical example consider the counting of test wipes of sealed radioactive sources; this is used to check for radioactive leakage. If all is well, the "wipes" should be at background level. How much above average background is significant? That is, when do we designate a source as likely to be leaking? The longer we count, the greater the level of significance we can obtain for the same potential leakage rate (maximum leakage rates are set by various codes). In this case counting time is opposed to the accuracy in identifying leaking sources. In general, the level of significance, also called the *confidence limit,* we use will depend on a value judgment that balances the effort of obtaining better statistics against the risk of making an incorrect decision. For most practical purposes one of two levels of significance are usually used; these are 0.95 and 0.99. A significance level of 0.95, or 95%, corresponds to considering significant those results that differ from the anticipated results by at least 2 standard deviations. A significance level of 0.99 is often associated with 3 standard deviations, although in fact only about 2.6 standard deviations are required to be significant at the 0.99 level.

> **Example 9-38.** A long-lived radioactive standard source gives an average of 928 counts in 1 min in a dose calibrator. It is a policy at our institution to make a recount if the count rate is significantly different at the 0.95 level and to call for service if the count rate is significantly different at the 0.99 level. If on a certain morning we count 999 counts, what should we do? For a 928 count $\sigma = 30.5$; a 999 count is 71 above average. This is $\dfrac{71}{30.5} = 2.3\ \sigma$; thus we should recount the standard source.

Example 9-39. A test film strip is sensitized by a standard light and developed each day as a check on a processor. The result of 10 days of normal operation yields the densities 1.13, 1.17, 1.15, 1.12, 1.14, 1.17, 1.13, 1.16, 1.15, and 1.17. What are the density limits if 0.95 confidence limits are to be used? First, we calculate the average and standard deviation; the average is $\overline{D} = 1.149$, and the standard deviation is

$$\sigma = \sqrt{\frac{0.0031}{9}} = 0.019.$$ The limits are $\overline{D} - 2\sigma$ and $\overline{D} + 2\sigma$, or 1.112 and 1.186.

The preceding examples illustrate statistical tests that utilize the standard deviation and the normal distribution. For counting problems and many experimental situations this is adequate; however, there are other tests that usually combine the standard deviation and an approximately normal distribution. In most of these tests a parameter is calculated and compared to standard tables; the best known of these tests are the χ-square, the Student's t, and Fisher's F test.

CHAPTER REVIEW

1. What are some of the sources of randomness?
2. Are systems that exhibit fluctuations always random?
3. How is probability related to the outcome of many events?
4. How are the probabilities of two discrete outcomes of the same event combined?
5. How are the probabilities of two independent outcomes of successive events combined?
6. What is the difference between combinations and permutations?
7. What is the *mean* of a distribution? How is it computed?
8. How is the standard deviation computed?
9. How are the binomial, Poisson, and normal distributions related?
10. What distributions are normally used in analyzing counting statistics?
11. What is a *significant difference?* How can this be different for different people?

PROBLEMS

Problems paralleling chapter examples

1. (9-1) The probability of rolling a 1 with a die is $1/6$. What is the probability of *not* rolling a 1?
2. (9-2) Find the probability that a light photon is *not* transmitted by a film of density $D = 2$.
3. (9-3) The probability that an x-ray is transmitted through a thickness t of shielding material is $p_t = 10^{-t/TVL}$. TVL is the thickness of a tenth-value layer. What is the probability of a photon being transmitted through three TVLs (that is, $t = 3$ TVL)?
4. (9-4) Use the model of the previous problem to derive the formula for the probability (p_a) that a photon will not pass through an attenuator of thickness t.
5. (9-5) In January a certain x-ray department took films for 5,392 views. Of these views, 279 required "retakes." What was

this department's probability for retakes in January?

6. (9-6) In 831 cases where radiopharmaceuticals were injected, ^{99m}Tc was the radionuclide for 786. What is the probability of ^{99m}Tc being used as the radionuclide in a radiopharmaceutical preparation?

7. (9-7) An ordinary card deck contains 52 cards. What is the probability of drawing a particular card—say the seven of clubs—at random from a deck?

8. (9-8) A sack contains seven red marbles and four yellow ones. What is the probability that a marble withdrawn at random will be red?

9. (9-10) A badly feathered dart is thrown at a 2 × 4 m board that has 20 balloons pinned on it. The balloons are 10 cm in diameter. What is the chance of the dart striking a balloon?

10. (9-11) Water contains about 2.7×10^{23} electrons/cm^3. If the photon interaction cross section is about 3.1×10^{-25} cm/electron, what is the probability of a photon interacting as it passes through 1 cm of water?

11. (9-13) A poorly aimed ball 4 cm in diameter is thrown at a picket fence consisting of 6 cm pickets spaced 6 cm apart. What is the probability of the ball passing through the fence without touching a picket?

12. (9-14) A total of 17 images are produced on camera 1 and 9 are produced on camera 2. Of these, 3 on camera 1 and 1 on camera 2 were gallium scans. Use 1 and 2 to designate the cameras and G and O to designate "gallium" and "other." Find $p(1)$, $p(1$ and $G)$, $p(1$ and $O)$, and $p(G|2)$.

13. (9-15) Black and white mice are used in a certain radiobiology experiment. An acute dose of 200 rads of radiation kills 15% of both groups. Are hair color and radiation death independent?

14. (9-16) Assume the sex of children is equally probable. What is the probability of a three-child family having all children of the same sex?

15. (9-17) For the probability tree in Fig. 9-3, what is the probability of a patient being assigned to room 2 with technician A and also having a bad film?

16. (9-18) What is the chance that a patient will be assigned to technician B according to the probability tree shown in Fig. 9-3?

17. (9-19) What is 7!?

18. (9-20) Cassettes 1 through 4 are stacked one on top of the other. What is the chance that they are stacked in order if they were positioned randomly?

19. (9-21) A class contains 6 students. If they sit in a classroom with 10 chairs, how many different combinations of occupied chairs are there?

20. (9-23) A certain patient dose is assayed in a dose calibrator 3 times. The results are 104.6, 103.7, and 103.9 μCi. What is the average?

21. (9-24) A certain unit is used for three different diagnostic procedures. Procedure "A" produces 4 views and is done on an average of 3.5 times daily. Procedure "B" produces 2 views; it is done 5 times per day. Procedure "C" is a single view; it is done only 0.5 time daily. What is the average number (expectation value) of views per procedure in this unit?

22. (9-25) The daily therapy doses for five patients are 100, 150, 175, 200, and 200 rads. The average dose is 165 rads; what is the standard deviation?

23. (9-26) Assume the probabilities described at the begining of the discussion of binomial distribution, p. 189, for mouse survival. If 3 mice are used, the binomial probability is described by $(p + \bar{p})^3 = p^3 + 3p^2\bar{p} + 3p\bar{p}^2 + \bar{p}^3$. What is the probability of 2 mice surviving and 1 mouse dying?

24. (9-27) If 1,000 cells are exposed to a photon beam that has a probability of killing $p = 0.999$ per cell, what is the probability that exactly 1 cell will survive?

25. (9-28) A tumor containing 5×10^9 cells is irradiated to a dose that leaves the tumor cells with an individual survival probability of 10^{-10}. What are the probabilities of 0 cells surviving ($p[0]$) and of exactly 1 cell surviving ($p[1]$)?

26. (9-29) A certain therapy facility averages 100 new patients per month. What is the standard deviation of this number?

27. (9-30) The film mechanical transport mechanism jams about 15 times per

month on a certain unit. What is the standard deviation of this amount?

28. **(9-31)** What is the probability of being beyond 2 standard deviations in a normal distribution?

29. **(9-32)** What is the probability of being between $\bar{x} + \sigma$ and $\bar{x} + 2\sigma$ in a normal distribution?

30. **(9-33)** A certain situation results in 100 cpm. What is the probability that a 1 min count will be outside the range of 90 to 110?

31. **(9-34)** How many counts are needed for 3% statistics?

32. **(9-35)** What is the standard deviation (in cpm) for a 5 min count at 2,000 cpm?

33. **(9-36)** What is the approximate range of oscillation for a Geiger survey meter with a 1 sec response time if the count rate is 100 cpm?

34. **(9-37)** Repeat example 9-37 for an information density of 400 cm^{-2}.

35. **(9-38)** The count following the one in example 9-38 yields 1,040. What response should be made?

36. **(9-39)** Another standard light (sensitometer) and processor are analysed during 10 days of normal operation. Test densities are 0.95, 0.93, 0.97, 0.94, 0.96, 0.98, 0.94, 0.94, 0.95, and 0.93. What are the density limits for 0.95 confidence limits?

Problems related to this chapter

37. If the probability of a certain outcome is 0.015, how many outcomes of this type should we expect in 200 events?

38. In a screening study there were 321 positive films out of 5,271 films taken. What is the probability of a positive result with this population?

39. In a certain study films were categorized as unacceptable, marginally acceptable, and fully acceptable. The probabilities for unacceptable and marginally acceptable films were found to be 0.08 and 0.34, respectively. What is the probability of fully acceptable films?

40. A regular tetrahedron has four equal sides. If it were used as a die and labeled 1, 2, 3, and 4, what is the probability of side 3 showing on a roll?

41. A folder contains 8 large and 11 small films. Because of their size each large film has twice the probability of being withdrawn as a small one. What is the probability of withdrawing a certain large film?

42. A certain type of tumor cell has a $\frac{1}{10}$ (or 10%) chance of surviving a dose of 100 rads. Assume that this is true for each cell in a multicell tumor. What is the chance that all the cells in a tumor are killed if the tumor is exposed to 100 rads and it contains
    a. 2 cells?
    b. 3 cells?
    c. 5 cells?
    d. 10 cells?

43. The probability of obtaining heads when a coin is tossed is $\frac{1}{2}$.
    a. What is the probability of obtaining two heads when two coins are tossed?
    b. What is the probability of obtaining at least two heads when three coins are tossed?

44. If the probability that death will be a result of heart disease is 0.4, what is the probability that death will result from other causes?

45. In how many different ways can 10 films be ordered in an envelope?

46. If there are 10 films, how many different sets of 4 films can be mounted on a view box?

47. A certain department has 10 technicians; they are not assigned to particular patients or areas. What is the chance that a patient will see the same technician for two procedures in a row?

48. Another department has 3 male and 5 female technicians. A patient is to have three separate procedures (1 technician per procedure). What is the chance that the patient will be handled only by female technicians? Assume each technician is assigned to one procedure only.

49. A certain physician has 5 cancer patients with very similar disease. He predicts that there is a probability of 0.6 of obtaining a cure in each case. Find the probabilities of
    a. all 5 cured.
    b. 4 cures.
    c. 3 cures.
    d. 3 or more cures.
    e. no cures.

50. A certain department has 4 technicians,

2 residents, and 2 machines. What is the probability that a patient has a particular technician, resident, and machine if one of each are randomly assigned?

51. Mrs. Jones has cancer but no one knows it. For her to be cured will require that she go to a physician, that the physician make a correct diagnosis, and that correct therapy be applied. If the probabilities are

Going to physician	$p = 0.6$
Correct diagnosis	$p = 0.7$
Correct therapy resulting in cure	$p = 0.8$

what is the probability that Mrs. Jones will be cured?

52. In the preceding problem, Mrs. Jones is going to a physician. What is her chance of cure now?

53. If the probability for unilateral breast cancer at age 65 years is about 0.001 (0.1%), what is the chance of bilateral disease if this is an unrelated coincidental disease?

54. Find the probability distribution for the number of heads appearing when four coins are tossed:
    a. $f(0)$ d. $f(3)$
    b. $f(1)$ e. $f(4)$
    c. $f(2)$

55. In rolling two dice, the probability distribution for the sum of the numbers is:

$f(2) = 1/36$	$f(8) = 5/36$
$f(3) = 2/36$	$f(9) = 4/36$
$f(4) = 3/36$	$f(10) = 3/36$
$f(5) = 4/36$	$f(11) = 2/36$
$f(6) = 5/36$	$f(12) = 1/36$
$f(7) = 6/36$	

Find the expectation value of rolling a pair of dice.

56. The ages for ten students (the students are called "A," "B," etc.) are:

A. 18	E. 24	H. 23
B. 32	F. 22	I. 20
C. 17	G. 21	J. 28
D. 18		

a. Find the mean age.
b. Find the standard deviation.

57. Dr. X biopsies suspicious lesions. For several years about $1/10$ of the biopsies have been positive. Each week he biopsies 90 people.

a. What is the average number of positive biopsies that can be expected in this group?
b. Using the Poisson distribution approximation, estimate the standard deviation for the number of biopsies.
c. Using the Gaussian results for standard deviation, estimate how often he will have more than 12 positive biopsies in a week.

58. What is the standard deviation in the number of counts if 100 counts are recorded?

59. A certain sensitometer processor-densitometer yields an average "middle" density of 1.13 with a standard deviation of 0.03. If the service personnel are to be called if the daily density measurement is beyond the range 1.07 − 1.19, how many calls can be expected per year (365 days) resulting from statistical fluctuation?

60. How many counts are needed for 0.1% statistics?

Objective questions

61. Out of every four patients with a certain disease, two will die, one will recover without serious complications, and one will recover with serious complications. The probability that a patient dies is:
    a. 0.25   c. 0.75
    b. 0.50   d. 1.00

62. For a nuclear detection situation that averages 10,000 counts, repeated experimental counts will be within the limits shown 68% of the time:
    a. 9,999 to 10,001
    b. 9,990 to 10,010
    c. 9,900 to 10,100
    d. 9,000 to 11,000
    e. 5,000 to 20,000

63. On the basis of a calculation it is estimated that a certain size and type of tumor will be killed in 50% of the patients exposed to a certain amount of radiation. If 100 such patients are treated in this way, the number of tumors killed will be:
    a. exactly 50
    b. approximately 50
    c. 0
    d. 100

64. A certain nuclear counter such as a GM counter is on for 1 min. It records 1,000 counts. The "standard deviation" of this measured counting rate is about:
    a. 1 d. 50
    b. 10 e. 100
    c. 30

65. The probability that an observed counting rate will be at least 2 standard deviations away from the average is nearest to:
    a. 0.01 d. 0.3
    b. 0.03 e. 0.95
    c. 0.1

66. Significance is a test between two hypotheses. The hypothesis that there is no effect is known as the _____ hypothesis.
    a. null
    b. random chance
    c. zero
    d. chance
    e. Monte Carlo

67. When a test shows that a certain hypothesis is "not significant," the best statement we can make is that:
    a. The alternate hypothesis is correct.
    b. The considered hypothesis is incorrect.
    c. More data might make the hypothesis "significant."
    d. There is not significance in the research.

68. For a certain disease, there are two types of therapy—methods A and B. Patients can be treated by one therapy or both. The probability of "cure" is:

no treatment	$P_0 = 0.00$
a only	$P_a = 0.30$
b only	$P_b = 0.40$
a and b	$P_{ab} = 0.58$

These probabilities are consistent with which of the following hypotheses?
    a. a and b are effective with different patients. None of those cured by a could have been cured by b, and vice versa.
    b. a and b have independent probability and independent modes of action.
    c. There is a synergistic relation, enhancing chances of a cure.
    d. There is a synergistic relation, depressing the chances of a cure.

69. An ordinary die has six sides numbered 1 to 6. In an honest roll each side is equally likely to come up. What is the probability that a 3 will show on a single roll?
    a. $p = 0$
    b. $p = \frac{1}{6}$
    c. $p = \frac{5}{6}$
    d. $p = 1$
    e. $p = 6$

70. A 10% difference between intensities in two pixels can be seen with 95% confidence if the pixels contain at least:
    a. 10 counts
    b. 100 counts
    c. 160 counts
    d. 400 counts
    e. 1,000 counts

71. The probability that the measured density in a sensitometer test is low for 5 consecutive days is:
    a. $\frac{1}{5}$
    b. $\frac{1}{2}$
    c. $(\frac{1}{5})^2$
    d. $(\frac{1}{2})^5$
    e. $\frac{1}{10}$

CHAPTER 10

Elementary calculus

Calculus is the mathematics of variable quantities. One parameter of a problem may be defined by its relationship to another parameter. If the first parameter changes in a specified way, the other will also change. Calculus is essential in deriving many such relationships in engineering and physics. Here we will mainly consider the terminology and uses of calculus without attempting to derive its basic formulas.

REVIEW OF FUNCTIONS

At its simplest level, calculus is concerned with the change of one variable when another variable changes. There must be a well-defined, functional relationship between the variables for any mathematical assessment to be made. The functional relationship can be expressed in several ways: as an algebraic function, as a geometric function (graph), or as a tabular function.

ALGEBRAIC FUNCTIONS. When the value of one variable (y) is determined by an expression involving another variable (x), we say that y is a function of x, or:

$$y = f(x)$$

For each value of x there is a definite value of y that, at least in principle, can be calculated.

GEOMETRIC FUNCTIONS. The relationship between two variables can also be defined by means of a graph, frequently a line graph; other forms are possible. In such a graph the horizontal axis usually represents the independent variable and the vertical axis the dependent variable (Chapter 6). For each given value of the independent variable, the graph shows the value of the dependent variable. We have discussed the concept of slope associated with smooth-line graphs. Calculus will be used to further refine this concept.

TABULAR FUNCTIONS. Functional relationships can also be expressed in a table. Consider the following trigonometric functional relationship:

$$y = \sin \theta$$

where y and θ are dependent and independent variables, respectively. The trigonometric tables on p. 104 express such functional relationships. To be useful for our purposes, these relationships must be reasonably smooth.

RATE OF CHANGE

As we mentioned, we can consider the change in the dependent variable as a function of the change in the independent variable. For example, the number of radioactive nuclei (dependent variable) in a sample will change with time (independent variable). The *rate of change* is the number of nuclei that change each second.

AVERAGE RATE OF CHANGE. The *average rate of change* is usually defined for a specified interval of the independent variable. It is therefore the ratio of change in the dependent variable divided by the interval (change) in the independent variable. Consider the case of a radon seed implant. In 24 hours the dose delivered to the volume of interest is 500 rads. The dose can be considered as the dependent variable; its change (ΔD) is the 500 rads accumulated during the change in time (ΔT), which is 24 hours. Here we use the Greek letter delta to indicate the change; Δ is read "the change in." In our case the average rate of change in the dose during this 24-hour period is $\frac{\Delta D}{\Delta T} = \frac{500}{24} = 20.8$ rads/hour. In general the average rate of change in the dependent variable y with a change in the independent variable x is $\frac{\Delta y}{\Delta x}$.

> **Example 10-1.** A capacitor-discharge x-ray machine has a charge of 0.10 coulomb at the beginning of a 0.1 sec exposure. At the end of the exposure the remaining charge is 0.08 coulomb. What is the average rate of change of the charge with time during the exposure? Here $\Delta Q = 0.08 - 0.10 = -0.02$ coulomb; $\Delta t = 0.1$ sec. The rate of change is $\frac{\Delta Q}{\Delta t} = \frac{-0.02}{0.1} = -0.2$ coulomb/sec.

The change in a quantity is the final amount minus the initial amount. If this change is negative, as in example 10-1, the quantity has decreased.

> **Example 10-2.** In passing through 2 cm of water, a beam of 40 keV photons will be reduced to 60% of its initial amount. Express the average rate of change as a percent per centimeter. The change in distance is 2 cm. Thus the average rate of change is $\frac{40\%}{2} = 20\%$/cm.

Several rates of change are given special names. Of particular importance in radiological applications is the change with distance in the energy of a charged particle, called linear energy transfer (LET). The electric current is the rate of change with time of the charge, and the flux is the time rate of change of the fluence.

AVERAGE SLOPE. With a smooth-line graph it is possible to consider the change from one point to another. Thus a change (Δx) in the independent variable is represented by a horizontal distance on the graph. The change (Δy) in the dependent variable is represented by the vertical distance between the

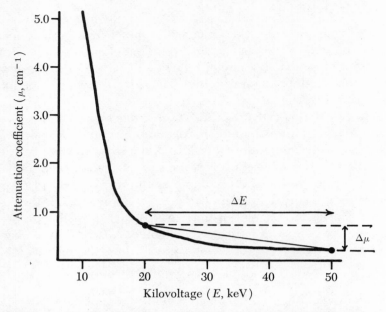

Fig. 10-1. Graph of the linear attenuation coefficient for photons in water. The changes from 20 keV to 50 keV are represented by ΔE and $\Delta\mu$. The change for both parameters can be represented by the straight line between the two points; the slope of this straight line is $\Delta\mu/\Delta E$.

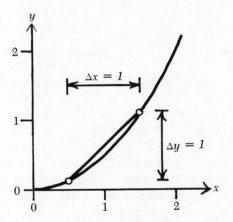

Fig. 10-2. Graph of the function $y = \frac{1}{2}x^2$. The changes between the two points ($x = \frac{1}{2}, y = \frac{1}{8}$) and ($x = 1\frac{1}{2}, y = 1\frac{1}{8}$) are $\Delta x = 1$, $\Delta y = 1$. The slope of the line between these points is $\Delta y/\Delta x = 1$.

two points. In the example shown in Fig. 10-1, a straight line is drawn between the two points; it can be seen that the average rate of change $\left(\dfrac{\Delta\mu}{\Delta E}\right)$ is the slope of the line.

Example 10-3. Plot the function $y = (\frac{1}{2})x^2$ from 0 to 2 and mark the points at $x = \frac{1}{2}$ and $x = 1\frac{1}{2}$. On the graph, indicate the values of Δy

and Δx as lengths; evaluate Δy and Δx numerically. This is shown in Fig. 10-2. Here $\Delta y = \Delta x = 1$, and so $\dfrac{\Delta y}{\Delta x} = 1$.

In general, the average rate of change between the two points on the graph is not equal to the instantaneous rate of change at either end of the interval. In other words, the slope of this straight line is usually not equal to the slope at one of the end points; the slope of the straight line is sometimes called the *average slope*.

A tangent is a straight line that just touches a curve at one point (Fig. 6-16). At this point, the tangent runs parallel to the curve; thus, the slope of the curve at the point of tangency is equal to the slope of the tangent.

THE DERIVATIVE

The average rate of change between two distinct points is given by the ratio $\dfrac{\Delta y}{\Delta x}$. If the points lie very close together, the average value will approximate their "instantaneous" values. When the points coincide (become instantaneous), the ratio becomes $\%_0$. To evaluate this ratio correctly requires a mathematical process known as "limits." A discussion of limits is beyond the scope of this text. For our purposes we consider instantaneous values two points very close together.

NOTATION AND MEANING. The average rate of change $\dfrac{\Delta y}{\Delta x}$ implies a change between two distinct points, (x_1, y_1) and (x_0, y_0). The *derivative* is the ratio at a single point (instantaneous value). To distinguish the derivative from the average rate of change a new notation is used; the derivative is usually written dy/dx, where d takes the place of Δ. The derivative dy/dx is read "the derivative of y with respect to x," or simply "*dy dx*." The form $d/dx\, Ax^2$ indicates "the derivative with respect to x" of the expression Ax^2.

As the points come closer and closer together, the value of $\Delta y/\Delta x$ will approach the value of dy/dx. For most practical purposes it is immaterial if we replace dy/dx by $\Delta y/\Delta x$ provided Δx is reasonably small. The average rate of change is conceptually easier to understand than the derivative. On the other hand, the derivative is mathematically easier to utilize.

APPLICATION. One of the most important uses of the derivative is in the theoretical development of concepts in physics and related scientific disciplines. For example, the decay of radioactive nuclei is often written as $dN/dt = -N\lambda$, where N is the number of nuclei, t is the time, and λ is the decay constant peculiar to a given radionuclide. The derivative is often useful in problems involving rate of change.

We will discuss the use of derivatives before presenting the methods of obtaining them. Thus, in many of the following examples the derivatives will simply be stated. The formulas used are presented in the boxed material on p. 210.

Example 10-4. The current i is equal to the time rate of change of the charge q. Express i as a derivative. The time rate of change of the charge is the derivative of the charge q with respect to the time t, or $i = \frac{dq}{dt}$.

Example 10-5. The charge q on a capacitor of capacitance C, discharging through a resistor of resistance R, is $q = q_0 \exp(-t/RC)$. The derivative of this expression is $\frac{dq}{dt} = \frac{-q_0}{RC} \exp(-t/RC)$. If $q_0 = 0.1$ coulomb, $R = 10^5$ ohms, and $C = 10^{-6}$ farad, what is the current at $t = 0.1$ sec? Use the result of example 10-4. The current is the time derivative, that is, $i = \frac{dq}{dt}$. In this case $i = \left(\frac{-0.1}{10^5 \times 10^{-6}}\right) \times$ $\exp\left(\frac{-0.1}{10^5 \times 10^{-6}}\right) = -1e^{-1} = -0.37$ amp, or -370 mA.

The derivative is equally important in graphic interpretation. Because the derivative can usually be expressed as a function of the independent variable, the slope of the tangent can be found for any point on the curve.

Example 10-6. The derivative of $y = x^2$ with respect to x $\left(\frac{d}{x}\right)$ is $2x$. What is the slope of the parabola $y = x^2$ at $x = 2$? The slope will be $2x$ or $+4$.

Example 10-7. At what value of x will the tangent to the parabola in example 10-6 be at 45 degrees? When the tangent is at 45 degrees, the slope $m = \tan 45° = 1 = \frac{dy}{dx} = 2x$. Thus $x = \frac{1}{2}$.

The derivative is useful in many other ways. One is in problems involving maximum and minimum values. In Fig. 10-3 a schematic function is plotted. The slope at both local maxima or minima is zero. If we know the derivative, we can use this condition to identify values of the independent variable that might be maxima or minima. Consider the curve defined by the relation $y = 1 - x^2$. The derivative of y is $-2x$; this will be zero when $x = 0$. Thus the maximum or minimum will occur at $x = 0$. That this is a maximum can be shown by evaluating the function at neighboring points. Since there is no other of x value for which the derivative is zero, we can also see that there is no other maximum or minimum on the entire curve.

Example 10-8. We wish to make a cylindrical lead pail with a total area of 1 m². The pail is to have no top; we want it to have a maximum volume of V. To solve this we must express the volume $\pi r^2 h$ in terms of a single variable; this is done using the relationship of the area

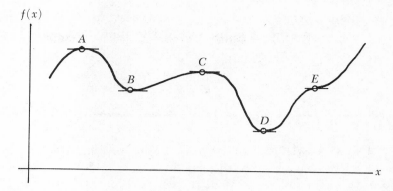

Fig. 10-3. Graph of a function with several maxima and minima. When a function is plotted, it may have local maxima such as points *A* and *C* or minima such as points *B* and *D*. At all these points the slope and the derivative are zero. The slope may be zero at other points, such as the inflection point *E*, but *must* be zero at maxima or minima, provided that the curve is smooth.

$1 = \pi r^2 + 2\pi rh$. We can solve for h in terms of r as $h = \dfrac{1 - \pi r^2}{2\pi r}$.
In this form, $V = \frac{1}{2}(r - \pi r^3)$. The derivative of this is $dV/dr = \frac{1}{2} - \dfrac{3\pi r^2}{2}$. This will be 0 when $\frac{1}{2} = \dfrac{3\pi r^2}{2}$, or $r = \left(\dfrac{1}{3\pi}\right)^{1/2}$
$\cong 0.33$ m and $h = \dfrac{1 - \pi/3\pi}{2\pi(1/3\pi)^{1/2}} = (1 - \frac{1}{3}) \times \dfrac{(3\pi)^{1/2}}{2\pi} = \left(\dfrac{1}{3\pi}\right)^{1/2} = 0.33$.
Thus the optimum container has a radius of 0.33 m and a height of 0.33 m.

Another use of derivatives is in approximations. If we know the value of a function at a certain point and the derivative of the function at that point, then we can approximate the value of the function at a nearby point. This can be seen from a consideration of the slope. Call the known point x_0, $y_0 = y(x_0)$. We want the value of y_1 at x_1. The average slope is $m = \dfrac{(y_1 - y_0)}{(x_1 - x_0)}$. The equation for the slope can be solved for y_1; $y_1 = y_0 + m(x_1 - x_0)$. Provided x_1 and x_0 are close to each other the average slope m is approximately equal to the derivative. If we designate $x_1 - x_0 = \Delta x$, we obtain the following approximation formula:

$$y(x_0 + \Delta x) \cong y(x_0) + \Delta x\left(\frac{dy}{dx}\right) \qquad \textbf{Formula 10-1}$$

This is a useful formula. As an example, consider the evaluation of the exponential $f = e^{-\mu x}$ for $\mu = 0.03$ and $x = 1$; the derivative $df/dx = -\mu e^{-\mu x}$. We know that $e^0 = 1$. Then

$$y(1) \cong y(0) + \Delta x \, dy/dx = 1 + 1(-\mu) = 1 - \mu = 1 - 0.03 = 0.97$$

Example 10-9. At $\theta = 0$, the derivative of $\sin\theta$ (in radians) is 1. Use the approximation formula 10-1 to show that $\sin\theta \cong \theta$. In this case $\theta_0 = 0$, $\theta_1 = \theta$, and $\Delta\theta = \theta$; also, $\sin 0° = 0$ and $\dfrac{d(\sin\theta)}{d\theta} = 1$. Thus $\sin\theta_1 \cong \sin\theta_0 + \Delta\theta\left[\dfrac{d(\sin\theta)}{d\theta}\right]$, or $\sin\theta \cong 0 + \theta(1) = \theta$.

DIFFERENTIATION. The process of obtaining the derivative is called *differentiation*. It is a process that can be carried out for any continuous function. To obtain derivatives, we will rely in part on the derivations presented in standard texts.

Derivatives of linear functions. First, consider the derivative of a linear function of the form $y = a + bx$. This function will graph as a straight line with slope $m = b$. Since the derivative dy/dx is equal to the slope m, the derivative is equal to b:

$$\frac{d}{dx}(a + bx) = b \qquad \text{Formula 10-2}$$

As a special case, assume $a = C$ (a constant) and $b = 0$. Now the function is a constant. Formula 10-2 becomes:

$$\frac{dC}{dx} = 0 \qquad \text{Formula 10-3}$$

This is not a surprising result since a constant does not change.

As another special case, assume $a = 0$, $b = 1$, that is, $y = x$. Applying formula 10-2 yields the result $\dfrac{dx}{dx} = 1$.

Consider now the case of $a = 0$ and $b = C$. Here $y = Cx$; y is a product of a constant and the independent variable x. The derivative is $\dfrac{d}{dx}(Cx) = C$.

Since $dx/dx = 1$, this derivative can be written in a form that suggests a more general form:

$$\frac{d}{dx}(Cx) = C\frac{dx}{dx}$$

This indicates that the derivative of the product of a constant and a function is equal to the product of the constant and the derivative of the function:

$$\frac{d}{dx}[Cf(x)] = C\left[\frac{df(x)}{dx}\right] \qquad \text{Formula 10-4}$$

Example 10-10. The derivative $d/dx(e^{ax})$ is equal to ae^{ax}. What is the derivative of $5e^{-3x}$? By formula 10-4, $d/dx(5e^{-3x}) = 5\,d/dx(e^{-3x})$, or $d/dx(5e^{-3x}) = 5(-3)e^{-3x} = -15e^{-3x}$.

Derivatives of sums and products. Formula 10-4 is the derivative for a special product, the product of a constant and a function. The formula for the derivative of the product of two functions must be similar to formula 10-4. If the product is written $f(x)g(x)$, we would expect a term in the derivative to be of the form $f(x)\dfrac{dg(x)}{dx}$. However, since the order of a product is interchangeable, that is, $f(x)g(x) = g(x)f(x)$, we could also expect a term $g(x)\dfrac{df(x)}{dx}$. A complete derivation shows that the derivative of a product is:

$$\frac{d}{dx}f(x)\,g(x) = f(x)\,\frac{dg(x)}{dx} + g(x)\,\frac{df(x)}{dx} \qquad \text{Formula 10-5}$$

Example 10-11. Use formula 10-5 to find the derivative of x^2. Here x^2 can be written as the product $x \cdot x$. This can be differentiated as $^d/_{dx}$

$$(x \cdot x) = x\frac{dx}{dx} + x\frac{dx}{dx} = x + x = 2x.$$

The approach of example 10-11 can be carried out for any positive integer power of x. The result is:

$$\frac{d}{dx}(x^n) = nx^{n-1} \qquad \text{Formula 10-6}$$

Although not proved here, formula 10-6 is valid for *any* power, including negative and noninteger powers.

Example 10-12. Find the derivative of $\sqrt{x}$. We use formula 10-6 for this. Here $n = \frac{1}{2}$. Thus $^d/_{dx}\sqrt{x} = \frac{1}{2} x^{-1/2}$, or $\dfrac{1}{(2\sqrt{x})}$.

Another useful formula is the derivative of the sum of two functions, say $F(x) + G(x)$. An example is shown in Fig. 10-4. The slope M of the sum and the slopes m_1 and m_2 of the individual functions are related as follows:

$$M = m_1 + m_2$$

These are directly related to the derivatives as $M = {}^d/_{dx}[F(x) + G(x)]$, $m_1 = {}^{dF}/_{dx}$, and $m_2 = {}^{dG}/_{dx}$; thus:

$$\frac{d}{dx}[F(x) + G(x)] = \frac{dF}{dx} + \frac{dG}{dx} \qquad \text{Formula 10-7}$$

Example 10-13. Find the derivative of $3x + 5x^2$. By formula 10-7 this becomes $^d/_{dx}(3x + 5x^2) = {}^d/_{dx}(3x) + {}^d/_{dx}(5x^2)$. Formula 10-4 can be applied to give $^d/_{dx}(3x + 5x^2) = 3^{dx}/_{dx} + 5^d/_{dx}(x^2)$. Finally, we can use formula 10-6: $^d/_{dx}(3x + 5x^2) = 3 + 10x$.

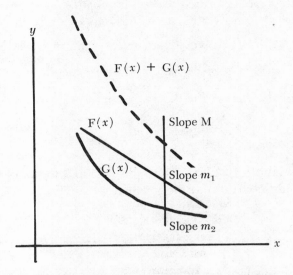

Fig. 10-4. Slopes of two functions and of their sum. The slope of $F(x) + G(x)$ can be seen to be the sum of the slopes of $F(x)$ and $G(x)$.

SELECTED DERIVATIVE FORMULAS

$f = f(x);\ g = g(x);\ C$ is a constant

$$\frac{dC}{dx} = 0 \qquad\qquad \text{Formula 10-3}$$

$$\frac{d}{dx}(Cf) = C\frac{df}{dx} \qquad\qquad \text{Formula 10-4}$$

$$\frac{d}{dx}(fg) = f\frac{dg}{dx} + g\frac{df}{dx} \qquad\qquad \text{Formula 10-5}$$

$$\frac{d}{dx}(x^n) = nx^{n-1} \qquad\qquad \text{Formula 10-6}$$

$$\frac{d}{dx}(f+g) = \frac{df}{dx} + \frac{dg}{dx} \qquad\qquad \text{Formula 10-7}$$

$$\frac{d}{dx}e^x = e^x \qquad\qquad \text{Formula 10-8}$$

$$\frac{d}{dx}\sin x = \cos x \ (x \text{ in radians}) \qquad\qquad \text{Formula 10-9}$$

$$\frac{d}{dx}\cos x = -\sin x \ (x \text{ in radians}) \qquad\qquad \text{Formula 10-10}$$

Derivative formulas. Besides these principal derivatives applicable to the simpler problems of differential calculus, there are others, particularly for the common *transcendental functions*—logs, exponentials, and trigonometric functions.

Several derivative formulas are shown in the boxed material on p. 210. They include the formulas already developed here. Various combinations of these formulas can be used to differentiate most common functions.

INTEGRALS

Integral calculus is in many ways the reverse of differential calculus, both philosophically and practically. Differential calculus breaks down a function into its instantaneous rates of change, whereas integration is putting the changes together to find the total change. Differential calculus speaks of "rate of change" and "slope," integral calculus of "totals" and "areas." There are two classes of integrals, the definite intregals and the indefinite.

DEFINITE INTEGRALS. A *definite integral* is best understood in graphic terms as the area under a curve. Consider Fig. 10-5, which shows the graph of the activity of a 10 mCi radium source in place for 48 hours. Because the half-life of radium is about 1,600 years, the activity of a radium source over a 2-day period may be considered constant. The "cumulated activity," a term frequently used in brachytherapy for radium, is the product of the activity and the time, here $10 \times 48 = 480$ mCi-hours.

For radon, with a half-life of 3.83 days, the approximation of constant

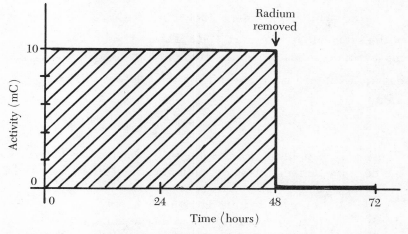

Fig. 10-5. Graph of the activity of a 10 mCi radium source in place for 48 hours. The cumulated activity corresponds to the shaded area.

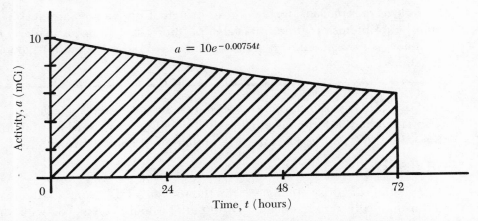

Fig. 10-6. Graphic representation of the activity of a radon source. The initial activity (a) of 10 mCi will decrease substantially in the course of a few days. The cumulated activity in millicurie-hours corresponds to the shaded area.

activity cannot be used over a period of days (see Fig. 10-6). Here the cumulated activity is still the area under the curve, but it is not equal to a simple product, as in the radium case.

There are various ways to obtain an approximation of the area. We can plot the function on graph paper and count the squares below the curve or we can plot it on construction paper, cut the area out with scissors, and weigh it.

The approach of calculus is to cut the area (mathematically) into small rectangular segments, as shown in Fig. 10-7. The segments have as height the dependent variable dX/dt in the figure (or y in the usual Cartesian coordinates) and as width a small fraction of the independent variable dt in the figure (or dx in ordinary Cartesian coordinates). The total area is the sum of all these segments. It is a special sum in that the width of the segments (dt) is not specified except as "sufficiently small"; dt is called the "differential" of t. The area of the segments in the usual x-y coordinates is ydx; to indicate the sum we use the symbol $\int$, which is known in calculus as the *integral sign*. The sum of the segments is shown as $\int ydx$. The interval of the independent variable must also be indicated; for the radon in Fig. 10-6 the cumulated activity for 3 days is written $\int_0^{72} adt$, and for the total output in Fig. 10-7 it is written as follows:

$$X = \int_0^{1/120} (dX/dt)dt$$

These are examples of *definite integrals*; they are equal to the area bounded by the curve defined by the dependent variable, the x-axis, and the upper and lower limits of the independent variable.

The solution of a definite integral presents various degrees of difficulty depending on the functional form of the dependent variable.

The simplest integral is the integral of a constant:

$$\int_{x_0}^{x_1} Cdx$$

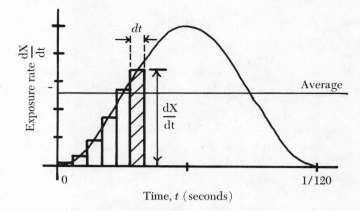

Fig. 10-7. Graph of the radiation output from one pulse of a single phase x-ray unit. The output rate, $\dfrac{dX}{dt}$, is approximately of the form $A \sin^2 (t/_{120})$, *where A is the maximum output rate*. The total output is the area under the curve. This area can be broken into many small rectangular segments such as the ones shown. The total area corresponds to the sum of all such segments.

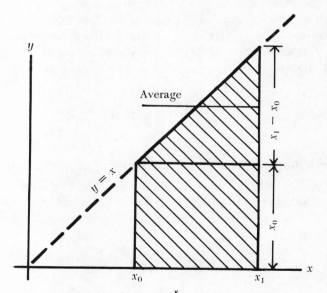

Fig. 10-8. Graphic representation of the integral $\int_{x_0}^{x_1} x\,dx$. The shaded area can be broken into a triangle of base $x_1 - x_0$ and height $x_1 - x_0$ and a rectangle of sides x_0 and $x_1 - x_0$. The sum of these two areas is $\frac{1}{2} (x_1 - x_0)(x_1 - x_0) + x_0(x_1 - x_0) = \dfrac{(x_1^2 - x_0^2)}{2}$.

In this case $y = C$ is the same for all values of x. The area is $C(x_1 - x_0)$. Thus:

$$\int_{x_0}^{x_1} C\,dx = C(x_1 - x_0)$$

A slightly more difficult integral is $\int_{x_0}^{x_1} x\,dx$. The function $y = x$ is plotted in Fig. 10-8. The figure shows the following:

$$\int_{x_0}^{x_1} x\,dx = \frac{(x_1^2 - x_0^2)}{2}$$

Formula 10-11

Example 10-14. Show that $\int_{x_0}^{x_1} Cx\,dx = C \int_{x_0}^{x_1} x\,dx$. With $y = Cx$, $y(x_0) = Cx_0$ and $y(x_1) = Cx_1$. Here the triangular area has base $x_1 - x_0$ and height $C(x_1 - x_0)$ for an area of $\frac{1}{2}C(x_1 - x_0)^2$. The rectangle has the dimensions Cx_0 by $(x_1 - x_0)$ and an area of $Cx_0(x_1 - x_0)$. The combined area is $\frac{1}{2}C(x_1 - x_0)^2 + Cx_0(x_1 - x_0) = \dfrac{C(x_1^2 - x_0^2)}{2} = C\int_{x_0}^{x_1} x\,dx$.

For functions that are positive, the definite integral is positive. For functions that are negative, the definite integral is negative. In terms of area the integral is positive or negative as the area is above or below the x-axis. If the function is positive for part of the range and negative for the rest, the integral can be positive or negative, depending on the relative magnitude of the positive and negative areas. For the same reason, a definite integral can be zero even though the function is nonzero for much of its range. As an example:

$$\int_0^{2\pi} \sin\theta\,d\theta = 0$$

The definite integral $\int_{x_0}^{x_1} f(x)\,dx$ represents the area between the x-axis, the curve $f(x)$, and the vertical lines at x_0 and x_1. An equal area could also be made by the rectangle with one side equal to $x_1 - x_0$ and the appropriate height. This height is defined as the *average* value of the function; thus:

$$\overline{f(x)} \times (x_1 - x_0) = \int_{x_0}^{x_1} f(x)\,dx$$

or

$$\overline{f(x)} = \frac{1}{x_1 - x_0} \int_{x_0}^{x_1} f(x)\,dx$$

Formula 10-12

Note that this is the average over the range from x_0 to x_1; over a different range the average would be different. Examples of such average values are drawn in Figs. 10-7 and 10-8.

Example 10-15. For the case shown in Fig. 10-8 and discussed in example 10-14 find the average value of the function $f(x) = Cx$ between x_0 and x_1. The integral is $\int_{x_0}^{x_1} Cx\,dx = \dfrac{C(x_1^2 - x_0^2)}{2}$. From formula

10-12 the average is seen to be $\dfrac{1}{(x_1 - x_0)} \dfrac{C(x_1^2 - x_0^2)}{2} = \dfrac{C(x_1 + x_2)}{2}$, as one would expect.

INDEFINITE INTEGRALS. If the upper limit of the definite integral is a variable rather than a specific value, the resulting quantity is a function of this variable. For example, consider the integral $\int_{x_0}^{x} x\,dx$. The results of formula 10-11 show that this is equal to $\dfrac{(x^2 - x_0^2)}{2} = \frac{1}{2}x^2 - \frac{1}{2}x_0^2$. The quantity associated with the lower limit is a constant. The value of this constant will, of course, depend on the value of the lower limit. However, the functional part of the result is associated with the upper limit. Frequently, in fact, the lower limit remains unspecified and the value of the constant is consequently not known. The sample integral could be written:

$$\int^{x} x\,dx = \frac{1}{2}x^2 + C$$

In this case the upper limit, x, is usually left out completely and the integral is written:

$$\int x\,dx = \frac{1}{2}x^2 + C$$

This is an example of an *indefinite integral*. It is called indefinite because the limits are not specified or because an unspecified constant, C, appears in the answer.

A very important property of indefinite integrals is that the function found within the integral is the derivative of the result. In other words, *the indefinite integration is the reverse of differentiation.* If $f(x) = \dfrac{dF(x)}{dx}$ then:

$$\int f(x)\,dx = F(x) + C \qquad \text{**Formula 10-13**}$$

This formula permits us to use derivative formulas to evaluate indefinite integrals. For example, since $^d/_{dx}\, e^x = e^x$ (formula 10-8), then $\int e^x dx = e^x + C$.

INTEGRATION. The evaluation of integrals is called *integration*. Some of the methods have been described in the preceding parts of this section. In radiology, integral formulas are used so infrequently that integration is best handled by reference to a collection of formulas. The boxed material on p. 216 is a rather restricted example.

Example 10-16. Find the integral $\int e^{-\mu x} dx$. This is just formula 10-19 with $a = -\mu$; therefore $\int e^{-\mu x} dx = -\frac{1}{\mu} e^{-\mu r} + C$.

SELECTED INDEFINITE INTEGRALS*

$$\int dx = x + A \qquad\qquad \text{Formula 10-14}$$

$$\int C\, f(x)\, dx = C \int f(x)\, dx \qquad\qquad \text{Formula 10-15}$$

$$\int \frac{df(x)}{dx}\, dx = f(x) + A \qquad\qquad \text{Formula 10-16}$$

$$\int [f(x) + g(x)]\, dx = \int f(x)\, dx + \int g(x) \qquad\qquad \text{Formula 10-17}$$

$$\int x^n\, dx = \frac{1}{n+1}\, x^{n+1} + A \qquad\qquad \text{Formula 10-18}$$

$$\int e^{ax}\, dx = \frac{1}{a}\, e^{ax} + A \qquad\qquad \text{Formula 10-19}$$

---

*A and *a* are constants.

For definite integrals there are two methods of solution. One is by using a definite integral table. The other approach is to find the indefinite intregal for the same function. If $\int f(x)\, dx = F(x) + C$, then $\int_{x_0}^{x_1} f(x)\, dx = F(x_1) - F(x_0)$. This latter form is sometimes written $F(x)\big|_{x_0}^{x_1}$, which is read "$F(x)$ evaluated at x_1 and x_0."

Example 10-17. The cumulated activity $\bar{a}$ for the example of Fig. 10-6 is $\bar{a} = \int_0^{72} 10\, e^{-0.00754t}\, dt$. Evaluate this. Since $\int e^{ax}\, dx = \frac{1}{a}\, e^{ax} + C$, $10 \int_0^{72} \exp(-0.00754t)\, dt = 10\left[\frac{-1}{0.00754}\exp(-0.00754t)\right]\Big|_0^{72} = \frac{-10}{0.00754}$ $[\exp(-0.54282) - 1] = 555.6$ mCi-hours.

CHAPTER REVIEW

1. How is the rate of change related to the derivative?
2. What is the difference between the derivative and the average rate of change?
3. What is the geometric interpretation of the derivative?
4. How can the derivative be used to find the maximum and minimum of a function?
5. What is a definite integral?
6. How do definite and indefinite integrals differ?
7. How are integrals and derivatives related?

PROBLEMS

Problems paralleling chapter examples

1. **(10-1)** An ionization detector measures

157 roentgens (R) in a 2.5 min exposure. What is the average exposure rate?

2. **(10-2)** For a ^{60}Co teletherapy beam the dose at 10 cm depth is about 50% of the dose at 0.5 cm depth. What is the average percent change per centimeter for such a beam?

3. **(10-3)** Plot the function $y = 1/x$ from $x = \frac{1}{4}$ to $x = 2$. Find Δx and Δy for the points $x_1 = \frac{1}{2}$ and $x_2 = 1\frac{1}{2}$.

4. **(10-4)** Power (P, in watts) is the time rate of change of the energy (U, in joules). Express P as a derivative.

5. **(10-6)** The derivative $d/d\theta \sin \theta$ is equal to $\cos \theta$ when θ is in radians. What is the slope of curve $y = \sin \theta$ at $\theta = \pi/4$?

6. **(10-7)** When will the slope of the line $y = x^2$ be equal to 60 degrees?

7. **(10-9)** The derivative of $\tan \theta$ (in radians) is 1 at $\theta = 0$. Use the approximation formula (formula 10-1) to find an expression relating $\tan \theta$ and the angle θ for small angles.

8. **(10-10)** The derivative $d/dx \, x^{1/2} = \frac{1}{2} x^{-1/2}$. What is the derivative $d/dx 5 \, x^{1/2}$?

9. **(10-11)** Use the derivative $d/dx \, x^{1/2} = \frac{1}{2} x^{-1/2}$ and formula 10-5 to show that $d/dx \, (x) = 1$ by setting $x = x^{1/2} \cdot x^{1/2}$.

10. **(10-12)** Use formula 10-6 to find the derivative of $d/dx \, (x^{2/3})$.

11. **(10-13)** Find the derivative of $1 + x + \frac{x^2}{2} + \frac{x^3}{6}$.

12. **(10-16)** Find the integral $\int \sqrt{x} \, dx$.

Problems related to this chapter

13. Find the average rate of change for the function $y = 2 + x^2$ from $x = 2$ to $x = 4$.

14. Find the slope of the curve $y = \cos \theta$ at the point $\theta = \pi/2$ (θ in radians).

15. Any smooth curve can be approximated by a straight line of the form $y = A + Bx$ for a short distance. Use formula 10-1 and data from Chapter 6 to find the constants A and B for the straight line that approximates the curve $y = x^2$ near the point $x = y = 1$.

16. Evaluate the integral $I = \int_0^1 x \, dx$.

17. Find the area under the curve $y = \sqrt{x}$ from $x = y = 0$ to $x = y = 1$.

18. Write in the form of an integral the aver-age value of $y = \sin^2 \theta$ for the range of θ of 0 to 2π.

19. The electric force on a particle of charge q is $F = -q \frac{dV}{dx}$. The V is in volts and x is the distance. Write an integral expression solving this for V.

20. A rectangle with the fixed perimeter p has a length l and a width $\frac{(p - 2l)}{2}$. Find the length l that maximizes the area of the rectangle.

21. Does the function $1 - e^{-\mu x}$ have a maximum or minimum?

22. In a radioactive series the number of daughter nuclei at time t is $N_1 = \frac{N_0 \lambda_0}{\lambda_1 - \lambda_0} (e^{-\lambda_0 t} - e^{-\lambda_1 t})$, where λ_0 and λ_1 are the decay constants of the parent and daughter, respectively, and N_0 is the initial number of parent nuclei. Use calculus to show that the maximum number of daughter nuclei will occur at the time when $\lambda_0 \, e^{-\lambda_0 t} = \lambda_1 \, e^{-\lambda_1 t}$.

23. The "stopping power" is sometimes called linear energy transfer (LET), or dE/dx (E = energy, x = distance). If a 6.0 meV alpha particle stops in 4.7 cm of air, what is the average stopping power for the alpha particles in air?

Objective questions

24. The derivative of a plotted curve at a given point is:
    a. the slope of the tangent line
    b. undefined
    c. a number ≥ 1
    d. the logarithm of the plotted function
    e. the inverse of the value at the point

25. For small values of x, the exponential function e^{ax} is approximately: $1 + ax$. What is the derivative $d/dx \, (e^{ax})$ for small values of x?
    a. 0
    b. 1
    c. a
    d. e^a
    e. e^{-a}

26. A local maximum or a minimum of the function $y = f(x)$ will have a derivative dy/dx equal to:
    a. -1
    b. 0
    c. 1
    d. either $+ \infty$ or $- \infty$
    e. none of the above

27. The symbol $\int_{x_1}^{x_2} g(x)\,dx$ can be read as "The _____ defined by $y = g(x)$ from the points $x_1, g(x_1)$ to the points $x_2, g(x_2)$."
    a. area under the curve
    b. average slope of the curve
    c. difference between the points
    d. value of $\dfrac{\Delta y}{\Delta x}$
    e. change in y

28. The function $y = \sqrt{1-x^2}$ defines the upper half of a circle of radius 1 centered at the origin. Use this fact and the well-known area of a circle to find the integral $I = \int_0^1 \sqrt{1-x^2}\,dx$. Its value is:
    a. π d. 0
    b. $\pi/2$ e. 1
    c. $\pi/4$

29. The "stopping power" LET can be written as $\dfrac{dE}{dx}$ (E = energy, x = distance);
    $\dfrac{dE}{dx}$ is most correctly interpreted as:
    a. the energy lost in a single event
    b. the average change of energy with distance
    c. the energy lost in traversing the medium
    d. the energy gain in a single event
    e. the rate of change of the energy with distance

30. If $\int y\,dx = x^2$, then y equals:
    a. 0 d. x^2
    b. 1 e. $\frac{1}{3}x^3$
    c. $2x$

31. The indefinite integral is normally written with a constant. For example, $\int e^x dx = e^x + C$. The value of this constant is:
    a. never of any significance
    b. frequently determined by "initial conditions"
    c. found by differentiation
    d. an indication of the uncertainty (standard deviation) of the result
    e. determined by more sophisticated mathematics

CHAPTER 11

Practical computation

For any given problem, we can obtain a correct answer only if we use the correct method, use a correct data base, and make no mistakes in manipulating the numbers. In this chapter, we will assume that our model is adequately represented by a mathematical formula or algorithm. Next, we must ascertain the completeness of our data base. For example, if we want to calculate the mass of an object from its material and geometric shape, we must know its correct density and enough geometric rules to determine its volume.

HAND CALCULATION

Virtually all mathematically possible answers can, at least in principle, be obtained by *hand calculation*. However, there are several problems: obtaining suitable "hands," the tedium of long calculations, and the high possibility of errors. In situations where hundreds or thousands of simple operations are required, mechanical means of calculation are invaluable.

The solution to many problems can often be found in more than one way. For example, if we are to compute $5 \times {}^2/_3$, we might first find the product 5×2 or one of the ratios, $5/_3$ or $2/_3$. For hand calculations, some ways are less tedious or error-prone than others, and of course we should choose the one that yields the correct answer with minimum effort. In dealing with multidigit numbers, most people find it easier to add than to subtract. Multiplication requires considerably more work and division still more.

> **Example 11-1.** Is there an easier way to solve $(4.72 \div 6.43) \times (5.76 \div 4.22)$ than straightforward calculation with two divisions and one multiplication? Yes. By writing the expression $(4.72 \times 5.76) \div 6.43 \times 4.22)$, you have two multiplications and only one division.

If possible, try to simplify the calculation by factoring and canceling. For example, to divide 100 by 36, divide both numbers by the common factor 4 to obtain ${}^{25}/_9$ as an intermediate step.

A special situation is presented by square roots in the denominator of otherwise simple fractions, such as $\dfrac{3}{\sqrt{2}}$. If the expression is written as $\dfrac{3}{1.414}$, a fairly tedious division is required. On the other hand, $\dfrac{1}{\sqrt{2}}$ is equal to $\dfrac{\sqrt{2}}{2}$ if we multiply numerator and denominator by $\sqrt{2}$. This changes

the appearance of the expression to $\dfrac{3\sqrt{2}}{2}$, or approximately $\dfrac{3 \times 1.414}{2}$.

Although this required one additional operation, the division is now simple and quick. In general, for hand calculations, eliminate the square roots from the denominator. This is known as *rationalizing* the denominator and is carried out by multiplying numerator and denominator by the square root.

Example 11-2. Rationalize the denominator in $\dfrac{7}{2\sqrt{3}}$. We multiply

numerator and denominator by $\sqrt{3}$ to obtain $\dfrac{7\sqrt{3}}{2 \times 3}$.

If the denominator is of the form $a + \sqrt{b}$, multiplication by $(a - \sqrt{b})$ will yield $a^2 - b$.

Example 11-3. Rationalize $\dfrac{(1 + \sqrt{2})}{(1 - \sqrt{2})}$. We multiply by $1 + \sqrt{2}$ and

obtain $\dfrac{(1 + \sqrt{2})^2}{(1 - 2)} = -(1 + \sqrt{2})^2$.

Errors may occur in any calculation. The purpose for which a result is needed will determine to what extent errors are acceptable. In radiology, particularly therapeutic radiology, a miscalculation may have fatal consequences; here errors must be kept to a minimum.

There are various strategies for reducing errors. Perhaps the easiest to apply is the *order-of-magnitude* approach, a crude estimate of approximately what the answer should be. For example, in calculating $21.57 \div 4.32$ we can expect a quotient of about 5; results such as 93.2 or 0.2003 are obviously incorrect. On the other hand, we cannot distinguish between the correct result 4.993 and one as slightly different as 5.243. For repetitive calculations of the same sort it should be possible to recognize the right order of magnitude of an answer, as in certain radiographic procedures where the milliampere per second (mAs) values are likely to be fairly close.

One of the best known checking techniques for additions is called "casting out nines." It can be found in most arithmetic texts. Two general checking methods will be described here. One is to reverse each step of calculation. For example, if we find the result of $21.57 \div 4.32$ to be 4.993, we can verify it by multiplying 4.993 by 4.32. Within the potential round-off uncertainty, the result should agree with the original dividend. This method is particularly effective in checking additions, subtractions, divisions, and square roots. Multiplication is difficult to verify, since the check requires a division. A second method, repeating the calculation, is less reliable, especially if done immediately after the first one. To avoid repeating errors, the second calculation should be carried out by a different person or by the same person hours or even days later.

Important in numerical calculations is the accuracy as measured in terms of significant figures or significant decimal places. In Chapter 2, accuracy was discussed primarily with respect to the input data. Here, we will consider its role in computation.

Most computation aids have an accuracy limitation. Computers usually have an accuracy of four to eight significant figures; most have higher ranges. Calculators are limited as to significant figures or significant decimal places or both; only a few have more than 12 digits. The accuracy of a particular operation usually corresponds to the number of digits in the display. Slide rules, once nearly indispensable, are now hardly used any more; they had an accuracy of roughly three figures if carefully used.

Graphic representations, carefully drawn, are accurate to about 1% of full scale length on standard paper. Tabular data generally have an accuracy of four, five, or six figures.

USE OF TABLES. In practice, we frequently need to refer to tabular data. An example of such an array is given in Table 4. There are two types of data. One is based on a *theoretical* model and, in principle at least, can be expressed as an algebraic function where the dependent variable is given for a series of convenient values of the independent variable. Tables of square roots, trigonometric functions, and logarithms belong in this category. The other type displays *experimental* (empirical) data and does not necessarily have an algebraic form. Much of the data used in radiologic applications are of this latter

Table 4

Exponential functions

X	e^x	e^{-x}
0	1.00	1.00
0.1	1.11	0.90
0.2	1.22	0.82
0.3	1.35	0.74
0.4	1.49	0.67
0.5	1.65	0.61
0.6	1.82	0.55
0.7	2.01	0.50
0.8	2.23	0.45
0.9	2.46	0.41
1.0	2.72	0.37
1.1	3.00	0.33
1.2	3.32	0.30
1.3	3.67	0.27
1.4	4.06	0.25
1.5	4.48	0.22

type; technique factors, depth dose tables, and radionuclide dosages are examples.

To be useful, tables must be applicable to the situation at hand or at least convertible. For example, exposure factors as a function of skull thickness would not be suitable for radiographs of an abdomen of the same thickness.

Tables must also have sufficient accuracy. Theoretical tables, such as for trigonometric functions, can be produced to any accuracy desired. However, as significant figures are added to both independent and dependent variables, the tables become bigger. Tables of empirical data, in contrast, are inherently limited by the accuracy of the observations.

Important for tabulations, particularly of experimental data, are the reliability and currency of the assumptions and parameters used. For example, a few years ago the accepted value for the exposure at 1 cm for a 1 millicurie point source of radium was lowered by about 2% as a result of new experiments and calculations. This required a change of the radium dosage tables derived from the older value. Outdated tables should not be used without correction.

Interpolation. Sometimes we need a value that lies between two table values. For example, we might look for $e^{1.25}$, a value not given in Table 4 but that lies between 1.2 and 1.3. An approximate evaluation for an intermediate point is called *interpolation*. It will generally work best if the underlying function is smooth, that is, if the graph of the function contains only gentle curves such as e^x or $\sin(x)$, and is most precise when the tabulated points are close together. *Linear interpolation* assumes that the function is approximately linear between the two adjacent points. Such an evaluation can be carried out graphically or by formula.

In a graph the function to be evaluated is plotted as a series of points, a straight line is drawn between the adjacent points, and the desired value is read off the appropriate coordinate (Fig. 11-1).

> **Example 11-4.** Use Fig. 11-1 to find the value of $e^{1.27}$. This can be read from the graph in the same manner as for $e^{1.25}$. Here $e^{1.27}$ is found to be approximately 3.56.

This example shows that *graphic interpolation* can be used readily for any value of the independent variable between two given points.

In some cases, it is unnecessary to graph the data for interpolation. Examples would be when only one value between two given points is needed or when a calculator or computer is available. In such cases, *algebraic interpolation* is to be preferred. For a value halfway between two given ones, we simply use the average. Thus $e^{1.25}$ is approximately $(e^{1.2} + e^{1.3}) \div 2$ or $e^{1.25} \cong (3.32 + 3.67) \div 2 = 3.50$. Although this differs from the graphic result (3.49), the difference is negligible.

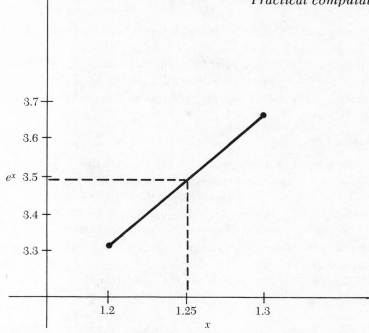

Fig. 11-1. Graphic interpolation to find $e^{1.25}$. The points for $e^{1.2}$ and $e^{1.3}$ are read from Table 3. The function e^x between $e^{1.2}$ and $e^{1.3}$ is approximately expressed as a straight line. The interpolated value for $e^{1.25}$ is then read from the graph as 3.49. This agrees to three significant figures with the exact value.

Example 11-5. Use algebraic interpolation to find an approximate value for $e^{0.55}$ based on the data in Table 4. The value of $e^{0.55}$ will be approximately the average of the values for $e^{0.5}$ and $e^{0.6}$, that is, $e^{0.55} \cong (e^{0.5} + e^{0.6}) \div 2 = (1.65 + 1.82) \div 2 = 1.74$.

For values of the independent variable other than the midpoint, we use another formula. If we define our known values of the independent variable as x_1 and x_2 (assume $x_1 < x_2$), the known values of the dependent variable are $f(x_1)$ and $f(x_2)$. Then for any value of x between x_1 and x_2, the linearly interpolated value is:

$$f(x) \cong \frac{[f(x_2) - f(x_1)] \, (x - x_1)}{x_2 - x_1} + f(x_1)$$
   Formula 11-1

For example, for $e^{0.55}$, $x_1 = 0.5$, $x_2 = 0.6$, $x = 0.55$, $f(0.5) = 1.65$, and $f(0.6) = 1.82$. Then $f(0.55) = (1.82 - 1.65) (0.55 - 0.5) \div (0.6 - 0.5) + 1.65 = (0.17) (0.05) \div 0.1 + 1.65 = 0.08 + 1.65 = 1.73$.

Example 11-6. Use algebraic interpolation to find $e^{0.64}$ from the data in Table 4. Here $x_2 - x_1 = 0.7 - 0.6 = 0.1$, $x - x_1 = 0.64 - 0.60 = 0.04$, and $f(x_2) - f(x_1) = 2.01 - 1.82 = 0.19$. Thus $e^{0.64} \cong 0.19 \times 0.04 \div 0.1 + 1.82 = 0.08 + 1.82 = 1.90$.

Formula 11-1 will also give results for values of x outside the range of x_1 to x_2. These results are known as *extrapolated* values. In general, unless there is considerable evidence that a function is very close to linear, extrapolated values are rather inaccurate. For example, if we use the values of $e^{1.4}$ and $e^{1.5}$ from Table 4 to estimate e^2, we obtain the extrapolated value 6.58, whereas its correct value is 7.39.

CALCULATORS

The advent of inexpensive hand-held *calculators* has been of great benefit in dealing with quantitative data. A major reason is the great saving in time. After you obtain a calculator, read the instruction book supplied with the calculator thoroughly until each operation is understood. Start with the basic four functions. Next find out how to "erase" or "clear" to delete incorrect numbers or numbers that are no longer needed. Chain operations are calculations that involve more than two numbers and possibly more than one operation. Learn how the result of one operation is carried over into the next operation.

> **Example 11-7.** Carry out the operation $3 \times 5 \div 6$. Key in 3 and the first operation, multiplication, then 5, and then the equal sign; the intermediate result, 15, should appear in the display. Now key in the second operation, division, and the last number, 6. When the equal sign is depressed, the result, 2.5, should appear in the display register. On some machines the intermediate equal is not needed and the intermediate result (15) will appear when the division key is depressed.

PROGRAMMABLE CALCULATORS AND COMPUTERS

The ultimate for computation are programmable machines. They range from small hand-held *programmable calculators* to the larger tabletop computers, "minicomputers," and large *computers*. Programmability simply means that we can tell the unit in advance what calculations we wish to perform. The program will then save us the labor of punching buttons. For example, if we have a series of numbers, each of which is to be processed in the same way (perhaps first divided by 5, added to 3, and then the natural logarithm taken) a programmed calculator will make quick work of this. Once programmed, all we need to do is key in each of our numbers and then hit the key turning control over to the program. The result of many steps of calculation will appear after a time without our further intervention.

PROGRAM OPERATIONS. In a programmable calculator the memory may contain not only numerical values but instructions as well. These instructions can be thought of in terms of keystrokes on a calculator. Normally, they are carried out one after another in sequence, called a *linear program*. On all but the smallest units there is also the capability to *branch*. At the branch the sequence of operations follows one of several alternate paths. Which branch of the program will be executed is usually determined by a numerical value (Fig. 11-2).

Not only does programming put emphasis on the steps of the operation, but there is an increased emphasis on storage. Because programming is usually only of interest in fairly involved computation, a considerable number of intermediate results must often be stored. Keeping track of these numbers is a significant aspect in programming.

A linear program involves bringing a number from some sort of input or memory into an active register, manipulating it, and finally returning it either to memory or to output. Coupled with this is the possibility of changing the process based on branching decisions.

It is often useful to represent a program with branches in a diagrammatic scheme called a *flowchart*. Although this technique became prominent with computer programming, it has been extended to many other applications. We will consider only three flowcharting elements: input-output, calculation or manipulation, and branching. Each of these elements in flowcharting is represented by a unique box shape, as shown in Fig. 11-2.

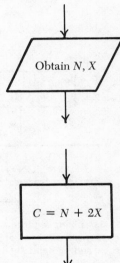

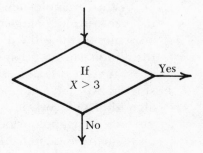

Fig. 11-2. Flow chart symbols. The uppermost symbol (the parallelogram) is used for input or output. The rectangle is used for computations. The diamond is used for branches. In the branch illustrated here, the "yes" direction will be followed when $x > 3$, whereas the "no" route will apply for $x \leq 3$.

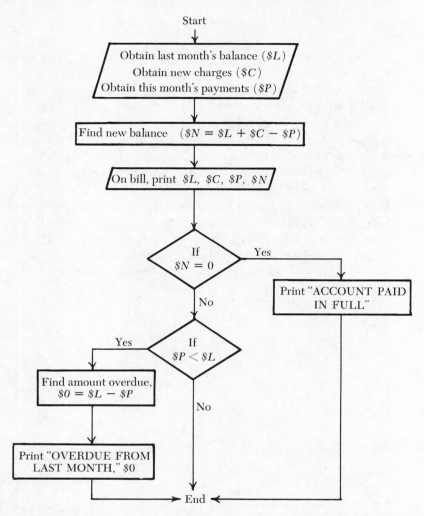

Fig. 11-3. A billing algorithm shown as a flowchart indicating input and output, calculations, and branches. Note that the computational technique to be used is not indicated; the algorithm can be processed by hand, by calculator, by programmable calculator, or by large computer.

A sample flow chart of a patient-billing algorithm is shown in Fig. 11-3. The term *algorithm* refers to the entire handling of the problem, including, but not limited to, the pertinent mathematical formulas to obtain an answer.

In this example new balances are computed and the old balance, new balance, current charges, and payments are listed. If no money is presently outstanding, the bill will also have the statement "Account Paid in Full." The institution expects payments to be made within the month. Thus if payments of amounts less than last month's balance are received, the difference is considered overdue and a notation to that effect is made. Notice that the sample algorithm will work on any device capable of carrying out the relatively unsophisticated operations detailed. That is, it can be used for hand calculations, on a small programmable calculator capable of the branching and printing implicit in this process, or on a large computer.

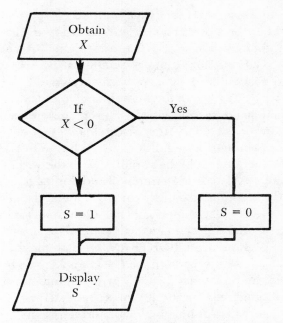

Fig. 11-4. An algorithm for calculating the "step function." The step function, $S(x)$, has a value of $+1$ for $x \geq 0$ and a value of 0 for $x < 0$.

Example 11-8. Make a flow chart to evaluate the "step function" $S(x)$ that has the values $S(x) = 0$ if $x < 0$ and $S(x) = 1$ if $x \geq 0$. Assume that x is read or keyed in. The first step of the algorithm is to obtain x. The next step is to determine the range of x the value falls into. Based on this result the value of S is set. Finally the value of S is displayed. The flow chart is shown in Fig. 11-4.

Programming languages. Computers with substantial storage capacity are programmed by means of a *programming language*. These languages are written at various levels of sophistication. At the lowest level is *machine language*, in which each step of the program execution is spelled out. This language is relatively difficult to handle from the programmer's point of view, because a large number of steps must be used for even relatively simple operations and the storage locations must be carefully remembered. Machine languages have the advantage that the programmer knows exactly how the problem is being handled, but they are rarely used for routine programming on any but the smallest computers.

One step higher is the *assembler language*, in which small groups of machine language instructions are handled by a simple instruction. This language is much easier to use but still tedious because of the number of instructions.

At the next level is a host of "user-oriented" *higher languages*. Whereas machine and assembler language are tied closely to the actual operations of the machine, the user-oriented languages are designed to match the way a person might formulate a task. There are FORTRAN and ALGOL for scientific problems, COBOL for business problems, BASIC for interactive programming, and many other languages with varying degrees of utility and power. A program written in one of the higher languages is translated into assembler or machine language instructions by a program known as a "compiler."

Programs consist of a series of *statements* that instruct the computer in the operations to be performed. For example the FORTRAN statement $X = A2 + B$ is an instruction to add the variable $A2$ to the variable B and store the result in a location X. At execution time, $A2$ and B must have actual numerical value. Despite the resemblance to algebra in some of the statements, such as $N = N + 1$, this is really just numerical; execution of this statement simply increases the value of N by 1. Each language contains many possible statement forms; as another example from FORTRAN, the statement IF $(X.GT.6)\ X = 5$ means that if X has a value greater than 6, then X is to be set equal to 5. These statements can be labeled, usually with a number, for convenient branching.

Once a program is written, it must be tested repeatedly before it is ready for actual use. This "debugging" will normally consist of three stages. The first eliminates those errors in programming that have resulted in statements unacceptable to the compiler; these errors become apparent when compilation is attempted. The second stage consists in the elimination of errors that result in a program "abort". The third and final debugging consists of a series of test runs comparing the results with answers determined in other ways. This step will uncover some of the more subtle errors that can creep into programming. Even when several successful test runs have been completed, caution must be exercised in any execution of the program.

CHAPTER REVIEW

1. What do we need to obtain correct answers?
2. Which method of computation is the most accurate?
3. Why may it be useful to change the order of operations in a computation?
4. Why is an immediate repeat of a calculation a poor way to check a result?
5. Why is the choice of computational aids sometimes determined by the desired accuracy of a problem?
6. How is the accuracy desired in a result related to the accuracy in the table to be used?
7. What is interpolation and why is it needed?
8. What is extrapolation?
9. When is programming worthwhile?
10. What is "flowcharting?" Why is it used?
11. What is a programming language? With what types of machine is it useful?
12. What is "debugging?" When is it complete?

PROBLEMS
Problems paralleling chapter examples

1. **(11-1)** How could $\dfrac{3.51}{2\pi} + \dfrac{7.42}{4\pi}$ be rearranged for more efficient hand calculation?
2. **(11-2)** Rationalize the denominator of $\dfrac{4}{\sqrt{5}}$.

3. **(11-3)** Rationalize the denominator of $\dfrac{(1+\sqrt{3})}{(1+\sqrt{5})}$.

4. **(11-4)** Use Fig. 11-1 to find an approximate value of $e^{1.23}$.

5. **(11-5)** Find an approximate value for $e^{0.75}$ based on the data of Table 11-1.

6. **(11-7)** Carry out the operation $(6.2 - 3.4) \div 5.2$ on a calculator.

7. **(11-8)** Make a flowchart for the algorithm to obtain x and then print x if x is positive or x^2 for x negative.

Problems related to this chapter

8. What is the best order of operations to evaluate $\dfrac{5 \times 21}{3 \times 43}$?

9. Rationalize the algebraic expression $a \div (1 + \sqrt{a})$.

10. If $y(1) = 1$ and $y(1.1) = 1.2$, find an approximate value for $y(1.07)$.

11. For $y(2.0) = 0.40$ and $y(2.1) = 0.44$, find approximate values for $y(2.02)$, $y(2.04)$, $y(2.06)$, and $y(2.08)$.

12. Use a calculator to evaluate the following:
    a. $4.2 + 6.3$
    b. $9.2 - 13.6$
    c. $43.6 \div 21.7$
    d. 19.2×13.6
    e. $4.34 \times 10^6 \times 2.38 \times 10^4$

13. Use a calculator to evaluate the following:
    a. $(2.52 + 6.44) \times 7.63$
    b. $(2.55 - 1.23) \div 2$
    c. $(7.31 \times 4.4) \div 3.25$
    d. $(4.32 \div 6.43) + 1.15$

14. Write an algorithm in the form of a flowchart to evaluate the average and standard deviation of six numbers and then test for the deviation of a seventh number at the 0.05 level of significance. See discussion of statistical tests (Chapter 9).

Objective questions

15. In multiplication by hand, the accuracy (in terms of significant figures) of the result is:
    a. usually limited by the input data
    b. always unlimited
    c. restricted to two significant figures
    d. restricted to three significant figures
    e. never important

16. Assume you are carrying out arithmetic operations involving five-digit decimal numbers with pencil and paper only. The operation that will take the most time and effort is:
    a. addition   c. multiplication
    b. subtraction   d. division

17. The best way to immediately verify an answer in a numerical calculation is to:
    a. check through each step
    b. reverse the calculation
    c. calculate the answer again
    d. do an order-of-magnitude calculation
    e. repeat it on a calculator

18. If $y(2) = 7.0$ and $y(3) = 9.0$, then $y(2.5)$ is estimated by linear interpolation to be:
    a. 7.0   d. 8.5
    b. 7.5   e. 9.0
    c. 8.0

19. The value for y at $x = 1$ is 1; the value for y at $x = 2$ is 3. The value for y (found by linear interpolation) at $x = 1.25$ is:
    a. 1.15   d. 2.0
    b. 1.25   e. 2.5
    c. 1.5

20. For a 10×10 field the back scatter factor (BSF) is 1.036. For a 12×12 field it is 1.043. For a 10×11 field the BSF is about:
    a. 1.036   d. 1.042
    b. 1.038   e. 1.043
    c. 1.040

21. The use of computers in radiation therapy will:

    1   Make calculations inherently more accurate
    2   Reduce the chance of arithmetic errors
    3   Soon be required by law
    4   Reduce the computational time for complicated treatment plans

    a. 1, 3   c. 1, 2
    b. 2, 4   d. 2, 3

22. A large computer can normally:

    1   Calculate very rapidly
    2   Solve algebra problems
    3   Derive new formulas
    4   Calculate with unlimited accuracy
    5   Calculate with a minimum number of mistakes

    a. 1, 3
    b. 2, 4
    c. 2, 3
    d. 1, 5
    e. 3, 4

Tables

Selected five-place roots

n	$\sqrt{n}$	$\sqrt[3]{n}$
1	1.0	1.0
2	1.4142	1.2599
3	1.7321	1.4422
4	2.0	1.5874
5	2.2361	1.7100
6	2.4495	1.8171
7	2.6458	1.9129
8	2.8284	2.0
9	3.0	2.0801
10	3.1623	2.1544
20	4.4721	2.7144
30	5.4772	3.1072
40	6.3246	3.4200
50	7.0711	3.6840
60	7.7460	3.9149
70	8.3666	4.1213
80	8.9443	4.3089
90	9.4868	4.4814
100	10.0	4.6416

Greek alphabet

Capital	Lower case	Name
A	α	alpha
B	β	beta
Γ	γ	gamma
Δ	δ	delta
E	ϵ	epsilon
Z	ζ	zeta
H	η	eta
Θ	θ, ϑ	theta
I	ι	iota
K	κ	kappa
Λ	λ	lambda
M	μ	mu
N	ν	nu
Ξ	ξ	xi
O	o	omicron
Π	π	pi
P	ρ	rho
Σ	σ	sigma
T	τ	tau
Υ	υ	upsilon
Φ	ϕ	phi
X	χ	chi
Ψ	ψ	psi
Ω	ω	omega

Mantissas of common logarithms

	.0	0.1	0.2	0.3	0.4	0.5	0.6	0.7	0.8	0.9
1	0.	0.041	0.079	0.114	0.146	0.176	0.204	0.230	0.255	0.279
2	0.301	0.322	0.342	0.362	0.380	0.398	0.415	0.431	0.447	0.462
3	0.477	0.491	0.505	0.519	0.531	0.544	0.556	0.568	0.580	0.591
4	0.602	0.613	0.623	0.633	0.643	0.653	0.663	0.672	0.681	0.690
5	0.699	0.708	0.716	0.724	0.732	0.740	0.748	0.756	0.763	0.771
6	0.778	0.785	0.792	0.799	0.806	0.813	0.820	0.826	0.833	0.839
7	0.845	0.851	0.857	0.863	0.869	0.875	0.881	0.886	0.892	0.898
8	0.903	0.908	0.914	0.919	0.924	0.929	0.934	0.940	0.944	0.949
9	0.954	0.959	0.964	0.968	0.973	0.978	0.982	0.987	0.991	0.996

*Other information in the text includes a table of key words in word problems (Table 1, p. 15), lists of special angles (Table 2, p. 62), trigonometric functions (Table 3, p. 104), and a table of exponential functions (Table 4, p. 221).

Answers to selected problems

CHAPTER 1

1. Negative
3. -4
5. 5
7. 20
9. -9
11. $^4/_7$
13. $^3/_8$
15. $^2/_7$
17. 9
19. $^3/_4$
21. 1,243.8
23. $0.5\overline{5}$
25. 0.125, $^1/_8$
27. 1.1
29. addition
31. 10^6
33. $5^1 = 5$
35. a. 8
    b. -4
    c. -8
    d. -11
37. a. 0.36
    b. -2.35
    c. 3.41
    d. 2.5
39. 12
41. 1.728
43. 0.95
45. $^1/_{1,000,000}$
47. e
49. d
51. e
53. d
55. e
57. c
59. e

CHAPTER 2

1. ± 250 rads
3. 3
5. 5.3

7. down
9. 0.91
11. 0.9773
13. 3.0×10^1 years
15. 0.02752
17. 2.74×10^5
19. 9.6×10^7
21. 1.9×10^{-2}
23. 1.1×10^{-28}
25. 7.0×10^3
27. a. 0
    b. 2
    c. 0
    d. 2
    e. 0
29. a. 1
    b. 0
    c. 1
    d. 1
    e. 0
31. a. 1.5
    b. 27
    c. 5×10^2
    d. 0.00
    e. -2×10^2
33. a. 59.2
    b. 0.0124
    c. -0.45
35. No
37. 3.0
39. d
41. a
43. b
45. b
47. b
49. c
51. e

CHAPTER 3

1. $d_0 + 200$
3. 1
5. $x^2 - yx + x - y + 5$

7. $(x + y) \div (y^2 + y)$
9. $C_t = f(T)$
11. $A = q(A_0, t, \lambda, f)$
13. 60, 60
15. 50, 10
17. $\dfrac{(5T_f + 2,297)}{2,655}$
19. $x - 2 = 2$
21. $B(A + B)$
23. $E = N/(nt)$
25. $S = ^4/_3$
27. $-2 \pm \sqrt{2}$
29. $n + (n - 5) = ^n/_{0.6}$
31. $-y - 2 > 1 - z$
33. 50, 47, 44, 38
35. a. $3a - 3b$
    b. $-a$
    c. $a^2 + 2ab + b^2$
    d. $3a - 2b$
    e. $2 + 5x - 12x^2$
37. $-4x = 4$
39. a. $x = ^y/_2$
    b. $x = \dfrac{(y + 2)}{6}$
    c. $x = ^2/_y$
    d. $x = (^2/_y) - 3$
    e. $\dfrac{(y + 1)}{(y - 1)}$
41. 0
43. $x + 4 - 7 = ^1/_2 x$
45. $\dfrac{n}{10} + \dfrac{2n}{10} = 36$
47. $^1/_3 x + 10 = ^1/_2 x$
49. d
51. c
53. b
55. b
57. d

CHAPTER 4

1. $47.25°$
3. $60°$

5. 616 cm²

7. 36 μCi

9. 10 × 25 cm²

11. 4.37 cm

13. 13 cm

15. 5 cm

17. 1.11

19. 25 kg

21. 935 cm³

23. 4

25. 0.825 R/hr

27. 0.0062 (steradian)

29. 330°

31. 270°

33. 0.0068

35. 13

37. 14 cm

39. 1.8 cm^{-2}

41. 5.9 × 10⁶/cm²−sec

43. 0.037 (steradian)

45. a. 36 cm²

    b. 40 m²

    c. 12.5 cm²

    d. 314 cm²

    e. 188 cm²

    f. 157 cm²

    g. 78.5 cm²

    h. 17.5 cm²

    i 7.7 cm²

    j. 43.3 cm²

47. a. 180°

    b. 120°

    c. 15°

    d. 135°

49. a. 64 inches³

    b. 0.33 m³

    c. 0.52 cm³

    d. 0.79 m³

51. d

53. b

55. c

57. d

59. d

61. e

63. a

CHAPTER 5

1. $\sin 30° = \frac{1}{2}$, $\cos 30° = \frac{\sqrt{3}}{2}$, $\tan 30° = \frac{1}{\sqrt{3}}$

3. $\sin 150° = \frac{1}{2}$, $\cos 150° = -\frac{\sqrt{3}}{2}$, $\tan 150° = \frac{-1}{\sqrt{3}}$

5. $-\cos 85°$

7. 0.9205

9. 23°

11. 11°

13. 6.2 mm

15. 5.7°

17. 37°, 53°, 90°

19. 5.7°

21. 3.85 mm

23. 86.7%

25. 0.62 cm

27. b

29. e

31. a

33. b

35. d

CHAPTER 6

1. $4\sqrt{2} \cong 5.7$

3. 63°

5. 7.7, 6.4

7. 12 cm

11. 0, 4

13. 4.1

15. 7.1, 7.1

19. 0, 0.05, 0.85, 0.95

21. $T = 94.53 + 0.10t$

23. c

25. b

27. c

29. b

31. a

33. e

35. b

CHAPTER 7

1. $a^6 b^5 c^2$

3. 2.0×10^2

5. $\dfrac{x^7}{y^5}$

7. $x^2 y^{-2}$

9. 4

11. $\sqrt[3]{108}$

13. $\dfrac{2\sqrt{7}}{7}$

15. 2.6458

17. 3.3

19. −3

21. a. 27

    b. 2

    c. 25

    d. 1,024

    e. 1,024

    f. 4

23. a. 1.00
    b. 2.72
    c. 0.368
    d. 0.135
    e. 7.39
25. a. $\dfrac{\sqrt{2}}{2}$
    b. $\dfrac{3\sqrt{5}}{5}$
27. a. $|x|$
    b. x^6
    c. $|x|$
    d. 1
29. 100

31. b
33. e
35. c
37. a
39. e
41. e

CHAPTER 8
1. 3
3. 1.643
5. -0.477
7. 8.13×10^4
9. $\log \dfrac{I_0}{I} = \dfrac{x}{T}$
11. $t = \dfrac{T\,(\log{^N/_{N_0}})}{\log 2}$
13. 1.099
15. output α kVp^2
17. $\log(^A/_B) = -\log{^B/_A}$
19. -1.284
21. 27.1
23. $^1/_5$
25. $t = \dfrac{\ln\,(\lambda_0/\lambda_1)}{\lambda_0 - \lambda_1}$
27. a
29. b
31. c
33. d

CHAPTER 9
1. $^5/_6$
3. 0.001
5. 0.052
7. $^1/_{52}$
9. 0.020
11. $^1/_6$
13. yes
15. 0.018
17. 5,040
19. 210
21. 2.7
23. $^{48}/_{125}$
25. 0.61, 0.30
27. 3.9
29. 0.14
31. 1,100
33. 0 to 255 cpm
35. service
37. about 3
39. 0.58
41. $^2/_{27}$
43. a. $^1/_4$
    b. $^1/_2$
45. $10! = 3,628,800$
47. $^1/_{10}$
49. a. 0.078
    b. 0.259
    c. 0.346
    d. 0.683
    e. 0.010
51. 0.336
53. 1×10^{-6}
55. 7
57. a. 9
    b. 3
    c. 16%
59. 18
61. b
63. b
65. b
67. c
69. b
71. d

CHAPTER 10
1. 63 R/min
3. $1, -^4/_3$
5. $\dfrac{1}{\sqrt{2}}$
7. $\tan \theta \cong \theta$
11. $\dfrac{1 + x + x^2}{2}$
13. 6
15. $y = 2x - 1$
17. $^2/_3$
19. $V = -\int (^F/_q)dx$
21. No
23. 1.3 meV/cm
25. c
27. a
29. e
31. b

CHAPTER 11
1. $\dfrac{(7.02 + 7.42)}{4\pi}$
3. $\dfrac{(1 + \sqrt{3})\,(1 - \sqrt{5})}{-4}$
5. 2.12
9. $\dfrac{a(1 - \sqrt{a})}{1 - a}$
11. 0.408, 0.416, 0.424, 0.432
13. a. 68.4
    b. 0.66
    c. 9.9
    d. 1.82
15. a
17. b
19. c
21. b

APPENDIX C

Bibliography

1. Kemp, L.: Mathematics for radiographers, ed. 2, Oxford, 1970, Blackwell Scientific Publications, Ltd.
2. Selman, J.: Fundamentals of x-ray and radium physics, ed. 5, Springfield, Ill., 1972, Charles C Thomas, Publishers.
3. Catholic Hospital Association: Mathematics primer for beginners in radiologic technology, St. Louis, 1966, Catholic Hospital Assn. Publishers.
4. Jackson, H. L.: Mathematics of radiology and nuclear medicine, St. Louis, 1971, Warren H. Green, Inc.

Index*

---

*Note: t following page number indicates information contained in table.

LEARNING RESOURCES CENTER
CLEVELAND COMMUNITY COLLEGE
137 SOUTH POST ROAD
SHELBY, N C 28150